Your Sexual Self

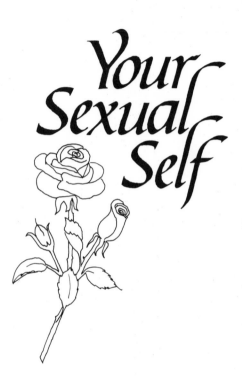

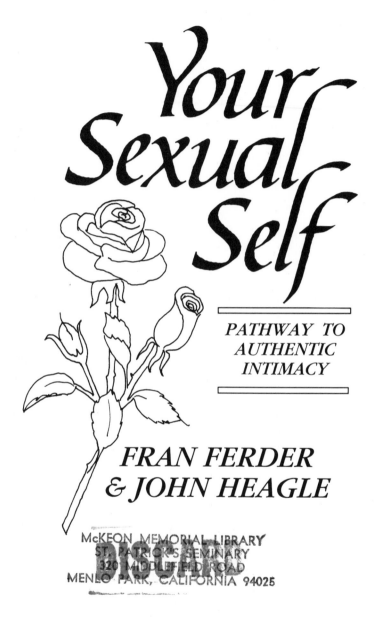

Your Sexual Self

PATHWAY TO AUTHENTIC INTIMACY

FRAN FERDER & JOHN HEAGLE

AVE MARIA PRESS Notre Dame, Indiana 46556

© 1992 by Ave Maria Press, Notre Dame, IN 46556

International Standard Book Number: 0-87793-479-7

Library of Congress Catalog Card Number: 91-77483

Cover design by Katherine Robinson Coleman

Printed and bound in the United States of America.

CONTENTS

For Judy Knight,
our colleague and friend,
who has helped us believe that
"each of us is entrusted whole
to our mother's womb . . ."

INTRODUCTION:
THE HUNGER FOR LOVE

A few years ago we facilitated a workshop on sexuality and human intimacy at a conference center in the Midwest. At the close of the weekend, one of the participants — a married man in his forties — told us there was something he wanted to say.

"This is going to sound strange," he said, "but this weekend helped me to name my pain. I came here with the feeling that something is missing in my life. Something important. The past few years have been difficult for me. I'm unhappy with my job. I'm angry with my boss. I'm disappointed in my kids. And I'm out of touch with my wife."

He paused for a moment, as tears welled up in his eyes.

"But this weekend, I became aware of a deeper pain. I realize now that the real hurt in my life is my fear of getting close. My wife and I have sex, but we don't have intimacy. We live in the same house, but we don't really know each other. I feel like I missed something when I was growing up. I don't think I ever learned how to express my love for people, even those nearest to me."

Without realizing it, this man had done more than "name his pain." He had given voice to something larger than his personal experience. He had pointed to an underlying hurt that exists everywhere in our society. He had found words for the silent ache that millions of people carry in their hearts.

The Deepest Hunger

In our work as therapists, we journey with persons who struggle with many different human problems. Some are wrestling with chronic depression, anxiety, or feelings of inadequacy. Others find their lives or careers to be in transition toward a new time and a new place. Some are seeking healing after becoming aware of abuse, emotional neglect, or addictive behavior in their family or personal background. Still others are trying to let go of their need for control, grieving their losses, or trying to face the anger in their lives.

But no matter how different these emotional problems appear to be on the surface, there is something they all have in common. Beneath the immediate issue, there is another reality that moves like an underground river beneath their conscious awareness. It is a tug of the spirit, a quiet fire that will not go out. This silent yearning goes by many names. Some speak of it as the loneliness of the human condition. Others use the biblical language of love. Whatever words we choose, the reality is essentially the same. In simplest terms, it is the *hunger for human relationships*.

This book explores the process of personal growth that we must pursue in order to fulfill this hunger for love. It examines human sexuality as the *energy of relationships*, the generative power that enables us to share the gift of authentic intimacy. More specifically, this book outlines the series of developmental tasks related to human loving — the physical, emotional, psychic, and spiritual journey that leads us toward maturity in our sexual and relational lives. It is intended to be a manual for understanding, a roadmap for reflection, a journal for the "seasons of love."

We are writing this book for ordinary people — people who hunger for love and want to deepen their capacity for authentic intimacy; people who are aware that "something important is missing" in their lives; people who know both the fear and the desire to "get close."

We are writing for adults who want to become more comfortable with their bodies and their sexual energy; who want to learn how to share their feelings more effectively; or who have encountered personal hurt in their sexual lives and are seeking healing.

We are writing for young adults who are preparing to make life commitments with a spouse, a partner, or a religious community; for husbands and wives who want to grow in their ability to celebrate their sexual union by expanding its energy into other forms of intimacy; for parents and teachers who are concerned about handing on an affirming view of Christian love to their children and to the youth of the next generation; for those who are celibate, whether by choice or by circumstance, and seek to integrate their relational needs in healthy ways.

In one way or another, this list probably includes just about anyone who is serious about personal growth. Most of us would like to be better friends and lovers. Most of us want to develop our communication skills and become more comfortable with our bodies. Most of us want to be more healthy and whole in our sexuality. If we are serious about lifelong learning, we want to deepen our capacity for intimacy.

Obviously, this is not the first book to address these important issues. What is distinctive about our approach? What further contribution do we hope to make? There are two ways in which this book differs from most other texts on human sexuality and relationships. The first is its focus on psychosexual development as the "soil" from which mature love and intimacy grow; the second is the biblical and incarnational spirituality that serves as a context for our reflections.

Psychosexual Development: Homework for Relationships

We are placing the search for human intimacy in the framework of psychosexual development. In practice, what does this mean? It implies that the ability to love doesn't just happen. Rather, it is the outcome of a formative journey — the flowering of healthy personal growth.

We are born with the hunger for human relationships, but the capacity to fulfill that hunger must be shaped and sculpted over a long process. It is not enough to have good intentions, personal determination, or religious conviction. The capacity to become intimate comes about only through a developmental process, a continuum of growth that begins before we are born and unfolds throughout our entire lives. Each of the stages of our growth — prenatal, infancy, childhood, adolescence, young adulthood, middle adulthood, and later adulthood, have their own relational tasks and developmental needs. In some mysterious way, each season of our lives depends on and flows from the previous one. The unfolding of our bodily energies, the emergence of self-awareness, the development of our ability to know and name our feelings — all these play a vital part in the process. If this journey is blunted, wounded, or traumatized in some way, our capacity for human closeness will not be fully realized.

Psychosexual development is another phrase for our pathway to love. It is literally "homework for relationships" — the deepest, most personal learning experiences and tasks that we must accomplish, stage by stage, if we are to become mature Christian lovers.

In the chapters that follow, we will reflect on each of these stages and their impact on our ability to be intimate and sexually integrated as adults. This is not intended to be a how-to book, although it is our hope that the information and reflections contained here will have practical implications for our readers. It is intended to be a journey of exploration and understanding, a way of looking at our sexual and personal growth that affirms the goodness of our bodies and the gift of human love.

Biblical Spirituality

The second distinctive aspect of this book is that it locates psychosexual development within the context of biblical spirituality. Our reflections are based not only on our experience as helping professionals, but also on our convictions as Christian believers. We are choosing to place these reflections in the context of a scriptural and theological vision — a vision that affirms the sacredness of human sexuality, the call to ongoing growth, and the centrality of love as an expression of Christian discipleship.

Obviously, it is our hope that what we are saying will be

helpful to any adult who is seeking to grow in sexual integration and human relationships. At the same time, we are aware that we bring our own formative experiences, our religious heritage, and our ministerial concerns into this endeavor. We are writing this book, therefore, especially for Catholic adults who want to integrate their personal growth with their spiritual formation.

Christians have long believed that "grace builds on nature." Our journey to wholeness and holiness takes place in the midst of life and involves all dimensions of our personalities. The purpose of human life and the goal of Christian discipleship are ultimately the same — to "grow in wisdom and grace" — to transcend our own personal needs, to love others in a life-enhancing way. "There is no greater love than this," Jesus reminds us, "to lay down one's life for one's friends." The approach to psychosexual development that we describe in these pages is intended to affirm this core vision of the gospel. In fact, it focuses on what we need to experience in order to "enflesh" the vision — the process of growth and formation that leads to and makes possible this other-centered love.

The purpose of human living is to lay down our lives for our friends. But we can't lay our lives down if we haven't taken them up. This book focuses on this vital task of *taking up our lives*. It explores our emerging self-awareness, our growth toward responsibility in relationships, our capacity to be intimate, the challenge to integrate our sexual energy in healthy ways, and the deepening ability to love in a mutual, life-giving manner.

1

COSMIC ALLUREMENT

Human Sexuality and the Origins of Love

In the beginning God created heaven and earth. Now the earth was a formless void, there was darkness over the deep, with a divine wind sweeping over the waters.
God said, "Let there be light."

— Genesis 1:1–3

The book of Genesis opens with two distinct but complementary stories about the creation of the world. Their literary styles and religious perspectives are different, but taken together they have become an important source for our theology of human relationships. In writing about sexuality, most commentators focus on those passages that deal specifically with the creation of woman and man (Gn 1:26–31; 2:18–25). The emphasis is placed on themes such as the equality and mutuality of the first couple, the fundamental goodness of sexuality, and the unitive and procreative purposes of marriage.

While these passages are important to the Judeo-Christian understanding of human sexuality, we want to begin our reflections by stepping back from this more limiting perspective to the wider horizon of creation itself. We want to view human sexuality from the context of God's first creative mandate.

Let There Be Light: The New Creation Story

"Let there be light." This is the divine command with which
the Priestly author begins his account of creation. What would
happen if we understood this mandate in a more personal
way? What if we approached this image not only as God's
first creative act in the universe, but as God's primal wish for
each of us? What if we heard in these words a description
of our unity with the evolving cosmos? What if we recognized in them God's gift of human passion — the energy
that stirs in our bodies and sets our hearts in search of the
beloved? What if we felt in these words the compelling call
to love?

In the late twentieth century a new creation story is beginning to emerge. This contemporary cosmology is transforming
the way we understand ourselves, our world, and our relationship to God. What is the source of this developing worldview?
Ironically, it is not arising from the reflections of contemporary
theologians, religious poets, or cultural philosophers. Instead,
it is coming to us from the scientific community, from the remarkable discoveries of this century regarding the origin and
nature of our universe.

What is even more remarkable is that these scientific discoveries share an amazing "resonance" with the vision of creation
that is portrayed by the theologian/poet of Genesis.

Let there be light. Most physicists now agree that our universe began some fifteen to twenty billion years ago with an
immense explosion of cosmic energy. This original "burst of
light" contained all the creative forces, all the elements that
would eventually unfold into star clusters, gas clouds, quasars,
and the sprawling galaxies whose immensity and numbers
are beyond our imagining. From that same primal fire there
evolved the mysterious combination of DNA molecules that
after billions of years leapt into life. The incredible variety of
life forms on our planet, the wonder of our bodies, the fire of
our passion, the miracle of human consciousness, the reach of
imagination, the power of love — all these are manifestations
of that original creative fire. They are literally "epiphanies"
of God's creativity — contemporary expressions of the primal
light.

Human Love: Light From Light

What does this "original fire" have to do with our ability to love? How is this primal energy related to our sexuality, to our desire to "be close" to other people? How can such a sweeping vision speak to us as individuals and to our search for authentic intimacy in the midst of our daily lives?

Poets, mystics, and lovers have long believed that "love makes the world go 'round." The newly emerging cosmic story seems to be confirming this ancient poetic intuition with new scientific data. The physicists of the late twentieth century tell us that the entire universe — from distant starlight to the whispered words of lovers — finds its origin in a common source. All forms of life and the systems that support it are the outcome of a primal burst of creative energy.

As believers, we name the source of this original fire to be God. The Nicene Creed speaks of the risen Christ as "God from God, *Light from Light....*" In the most profound sense, every woman and man — and indeed all of creation — participates in the second part of this statement of faith. Everything that is finds its origin in the brilliance of God's creative act. Each of us is literally "light from Light." We are energy from Energy, love from Love, fire from Fire.

The divine fire of love manifests itself in the most ordinary of ways in our daily lives. It is present in the warm hug of a friend or in the mutual gaze of lovers. It shines in the eyes of parents as they hold their newborn child. We see it in the faces of our sons or daughters when they announce that they are engaged to be married. It is the quiet radiance on the countenance of those who have journeyed into the mystery of contemplative prayer. We notice it in the presence of generative ministers and helping professionals who "lay down their lives for their friends."

Let there be light. The source of this embodied energy, the origin of this passion and compassion, is in God, and in that "first light" — the creative fire at the dawn of creation. Perhaps this is what the Song of Songs is hinting at when it describes human love as "a flame of God" and reminds us that neither death nor the dark waters will ever extinguish it (Sg 8:6f).

Cosmic Allurement

The presence of the divine fire is manifest in another way in our world. It shows itself as an energy of connection, the mysterious "magnetism" that permeates our cosmos on all levels of being.

In his book *A Brief History of Time*, the world renowned physicist Stephen Hawking speaks of the "four forces" that have been at work from the first moments of the creative fire.[1] The most apparent of these forces is the one that we call "gravity." The "law of gravity" is simply an evolving mathematical hypothesis that attempts to describe a mystery that is ultimately beyond our comprehension. That mystery has to do with the power of *attraction* that appears everywhere in our universe. Mathematics can describe this phenomenon, but it cannot explain it. Years after Isaac Newton wrote out his equations, he was still asking himself: "Whence is it that the sun and the planets gravitate toward one another?"

It is unlikely that science will ever discover a final answer to Newton's question or Einstein's refinements of his question; for beyond our equations there is always more mystery. In actuality, the law of gravity is simply another way of speaking about the "energy of attraction" that can be found at all levels of reality — from quasars to quarks, from the music of the spheres to the longing of human hearts. Cosmologist Brian Swimme has coined an imaginative word for this universal binding energy. He calls it "cosmic allurement."[2]

We human beings give a more familiar name to this "binding energy." We call it *love*. Love is cosmic allurement as it is revealed in our human lives and relationships. "Love is a word that points to this alluring activity in the cosmos. This primal dynamism awakens the communities of atoms, galaxies, stars, families, nations, persons, ecosystems, oceans, and stellar systems. Love ignites being."[3] In our human experience this cosmic allurement becomes conscious and intentional. Our sexual energy is an "embodiment" of the relational power that permeates the universe.

Teilhard de Chardin refers to humanity as "the arrow of evolution." In the emergence of self-consciousness and freedom he sees the unfolding of God's creative fire reaching another level of growth and expression.

What implications does this have for our sexuality and for the ways in which our relationships "embody" the mystery of cosmic allurement? In the development of our bodies and the growth of our inwardness, each of us, in some mysterious way, sums up and carries forward the history of humanity and of creation. There is a biological principle that states that "ontogeny recapitulates phylogeny." This is scientific language for something that is at once simple and stunning. In more understandable terms, it means that the growth cycle of the individual mirrors or "repeats" the history of the entire species. In our development, each of us is like "an instant replay" of the evolution of humanity and, at a more expansive level, of the history of the universe.

We can observe this phenomenon by studying prenatal development in human beings. In the early stages of fetal growth we pass through a fish-like stage with structures that resemble embryonic gill-arches between the eye and the forelimb. At this early stage of fetal development it is difficult to tell one species of vertebrate from another.

What a wondrous encounter with divine creativity! The history of each of our bodies is like a microcosmic summary of the vast story of creation. In his writings on marriage, Pope John Paul II speaks of this "inherent language" of the human body.[4] He describes the way in which each of us images the source from which we came. The direction and shape of our physical and sexual growth are a powerful reminder of our sacred roots in the evolution of life. In every human person there is an actualization of what Teilhard calls "the irreplaceably precious." It is a pattern that points beyond itself — to our ultimate origin in the divine fire, the light of God at the dawn of creation.

The Search for the Beloved

This pattern is found not only on the physical level of our growth, but also in the psychic and spiritual dimensions of our lives. The history of spirituality and the discoveries of depth psychology give ample evidence that we inherit and carry forward something of the inwardness or the "within" of evolution. We need only look to our shared world of symbols, guiding archetypes, and cultural myths to see evidence of this. In our personal dream life and the creativity of our unconscious we gain access to humanity's past psychic unfolding.

Is there an underlying pattern in our dreams and myths? Is there a story behind all our stories? Obviously there is a rich variety of themes, but beneath all of them, like a recurring melody, is the *quest for union*, for love. On the psychic level, as on the biological level, the energy of attraction is central to human experience. Cosmic allurement is encoded into our genes; the desire to reach out to the other is integral to our being.

On the psychic level this is often revealed through our feelings of spiritual longing. In all the great religious traditions, the central theme, the guiding passion, is the deep yearning for what Jean Houston calls "the Beloved of the soul."[5] In the course of our lives, this profound longing finds nourishment in healthy parental love; it thrives in the world of youthful belonging; it ignites into flame in romantic love; it deepens into enduring, covenantal friendship. But ultimately, the restless human heart continues to yearn for the Source — the Light from which all other light is derived. "In you is the source of life," the psalmist prays, "and in your light we see light" (Ps 36:9).

Let There Be Passion

Here, on the vast horizon of "continuing creation," we want to situate our reflections on psychosexual development. It is in the dialogue between the ancient biblical vision and the newly emerging cosmic story that the deeper significance of our psychosexual energy reveals itself.

Let there be light. Light is the biblical metaphor for divine creativity, for God's *passion* to share being. It is a word that expresses the generative act of God at the dawn of creation, the explosion into time of divine love.

Let there be light. It is a poetic and theological way of saying: Let the universe unfold. Let there be the radiance of a sunrise, the brilliance of summer lightning, the glow of distant stars, the sunny smile of friends, the warm embrace of lovers. Let there be energy. Let there be the belching of volcanoes, the dance of the Northern Lights, the leaping flames of campfires, the racing heartbeat, the delight of the beloved.

Let there be passion. Let there be prophetic zeal, creative imagination, fiery conviction. Let there be the ritual of courtship, the pursuit of romance, the ardor of lovemaking, the silent, shared flame of those who have loved long and well.

Let there be light. There is but one divine source of all these forms of energy. It is the same creative fire that brings flesh and bone, bodies and emotion, imagination and passion, love and mutuality into being. In the scriptures, light is a personal as well as a cosmic energy. It is an image for what the ancient Hebrews called the *kabod Yahweh* — "the glory of God." It is the radiant presence of God in the night of freedom, the flaming pillar that illumined the pathway toward a desert covenant, the luminous cloud that transformed slaves into liberated people, the transfiguring energy that shone from the face of Jesus on the mountaintop.

Perhaps it is this last image — the shining countenance of Jesus — that comes closest to personalizing the creative fire of God in our bodies and our relationships. That divine energy is within each of us.

In the beginning is the creative fire, the light from the Light. In the beginning is allurement, the divine power of attraction. In the beginning is relationship, the energy of love.

2

A FUTURE WITH HOPE

Listening to Our Psychosexual Story

For surely I know the plans I have for you, says the Lord,
plans for your welfare and not for harm, to give you a
future with hope.

— Jeremiah 29:11

These encouraging words are found in a letter that Jeremiah
wrote to his fellow citizens shortly after they had been deported from their homeland into Babylon. His letter was
intended to buoy up the hopes of an exiled people — a people
who wondered if this time God had indeed abandoned them.
Through the prophet, the Lord invited them to be patient and
reassured them of "a future with hope."

Whether or not we have ever been physically deported to
another land, there are times in most of our lives when we
feel *exiled* — cut off from our feelings, alienated from those
we love, uncomfortable with our bodies, guilt-ridden about
something in our past.

Few dimensions of our lives appear to be as vulnerable to
feelings of alienation and shame as that of our sexuality and
our search for intimacy. There are some obvious reasons for
this. Our sexual feelings are intensely personal and private;
they come from the center of our selves as embodied persons.
In addition, since the search for intimacy can only take place
in the context of trust, it also involves risk. It is not surprising,

21

then, that our attempts to be close to others can sometimes result in feelings of "emotional exile" rather than comforting mutuality.

In the difficult moments of our lives, we can usually look to our religious beliefs and practices for consolation. This is not necessarily the case, however, when it comes to sexuality. For some reason, the call to ethical accountability can quickly turn into harsh moral indictment in this aspect of our lives. Instead of being a source of healing and forgiveness, our religious heritage can sometimes leave us feeling ashamed and unworthy.

Is there a way we can overcome this feeling of being exiled from ourselves, from others, and from God? How can we maintain a genuine sense of personal responsibility without falling into self-recrimination? How can we reclaim the plans that God has for us — plans for our welfare and not for harm?

In this chapter we want to suggest a way of moving toward these goals by listening to and reverencing our psychosexual story. It requires that we stand before our lives with an attitude of self-acceptance rather than self-recrimination. It invites us to reaffirm the creative intention of the God who gifted us with sexuality in the first place.

Celie's Story: A Future With Hope

In her Pulitzer prize-winning novel *The Color Purple*, Alice Walker tells the story of a young black woman, Celie, and her long journey from brokenness toward healing. During her childhood and adolescence, Celie repeatedly endures the trauma of verbal, emotional, physical, and sexual abuse. Her self-esteem and her sense of uniqueness are badly damaged. She is sexually exploited by her father and by other men in her life.

But beneath Celie's pain there is a powerful resilience, an indomitable spirit that refuses to give up. Strengthened by the love that she has for her sister, Nettie, who is taken from her when they are young, Celie continues to seek for wholeness in the midst of her broken world.

One of the turning points for Celie is a friendship that

develops between herself and Shug — a woman who is as vibrantly alive as she is sensuously beautiful. In one of the novel's most engaging scenes, Celie and Shug have a conversation about God and sexuality. Disillusioned with her life and its pain, Celie has stopped writing to God because "he is just like all the other mens I know — low down, forgitful, and cheatin." Shug begins to tell Celie how her understanding of God has changed over the years from the "old white man up in the sky" to an energizing presence at the heart of life. Celie describes the ensuing conversation in these words:

> Shug a beautiful something, let me tell you. She frown a little, look out cross the yard, lean back in her chair, look like a big rose.
>
> She say, My first step from the old white man was trees. Then air. Then birds. Then other people. But one day when I was sitting quiet and feeling like a motherless child, which I was, it come to me: that feeling of being part of everything, not separate at all. I laughed and I cried and I run all around the house. I knew just what it was. In fact, when it happen, you can't miss it. It sort of like you know what, she say, grinning and rubbing high up on my thigh.
>
> *Shug!* I say.
>
> Oh, she say. God love all them feelings. That's some of the best stuff God did. And when you know God loves 'em you enjoys 'em a lot more. You can just relax, go with everything that's going, and praise God by liking what you like.
>
> God don't think it dirty? I ast.
>
> Naw, she say. God made it. Listen, God love everything you love — and a mess of stuff you don't. But more than anything else, God love admiration.
>
> You saying God vain? I ast.
>
> Naw, she say. Not vain, just wanting to share a good thing.[6]

There is a wisdom in this conversation that is both earthy and profound. Shug's homespun theology captures the vital bond between God and life, between the holy and the human.

But what makes this scene especially powerful is that these two women are sharing the deepest, most personal dimensions of their lives — their experience of God and their sexuality. They are entering into, listening to, and naming the underlying story of their lives, not just events linked by circumstances, but the deep, inner story of their search for the divine and their hunger for love.

Our Psychosexual Story

Our lives hold many stories. We have a family story, an educational story, a faith story, and a health story. We have a work story, a crisis story, and a creativity story.

We also have a *psychosexual* story. This dimension of our personal history involves the mysterious convergence of circumstances, events, experiences, and choices that have brought us to our present stage of integration or woundedness. Our psychosexual story contains all the moments of growth, excitement, discovery, pain, struggle, and questioning in our relational lives. This is the story of our growing up — our journey toward friendship and human communion. It is the story of our physical and emotional awakenings, our yearnings and our fantasies, our soaring feelings and our broken hearts, our desires and our dependencies, our struggles with shame and our breakthroughs to mutuality.

Like Celie and Shug, each of us grows up with a desire to connect: to find safety, nourishment, and protection when we are infants; to discover playmates and friends when we are in school; to choose a way of life, which includes the significant person or persons who will be our companions. These people become a vital part of the way we walk through time. Some, like our families, may be part of our entire journey in one way or another. Others enter our story at certain significant times as classmates, friends, fellow workers, colleagues, or lovers, and then they disappear. Still others — usually only a few — are in some way bonded to us through the most important times of our growing and changing. They are the real life companions, the "significant others" who know our hearts and love us in our weaknesses as well as our gifts.

The Importance of Our Psychosexual Story

What does our psychosexual story have to do with healthy development? Why should we spend time exploring these memories and messages? How will this help us to become more integrated in our relational lives?

The answer to these questions has to do with the importance of self-knowledge and self-acceptance in our journey toward integration. Whether or not we are aware of it, our sexual and relational history exerts a powerful influence on our self-esteem. And our self-worth, in turn, affects our capacity for friendship, our style of interacting with others, and our way of relating to God.

Our psychosexual story is like an emotional "memory bank" that stores all the events and experiences related to our relational development from our earliest moments of life. Its data is stored both in our conscious memory and in our unconscious mind. This vital flow of experience is also traced out in our physical self as "body memories."

Becoming more comfortable with our psychosexual story marks the difference between responsible awareness and psychic denial, between living in the light or hiding in the dark. When we know our story, we can begin to heal our past, embrace our present, and shape our future. With Celie and Shug as models of courage and honesty, we invite our readers to begin a journey of remembering and reflecting, a quiet trek into the world of understanding and healing. We will examine four important tasks in relationship to our psychosexual story: (1) approaching our story with reverence, (2) listening to our story with trust, (3) naming the messages in our psychosexual story, and (4) reimaging or reinterpreting our psychosexual story with healing and hope.

Approaching Our Psychosexual Story with Reverence

Our sexuality is close to the core of our being. In some mysterious way, it shapes our identity as human persons and conveys something about the way in which each of us is an *imago Dei* — an image of a loving and creative God. Perhaps this is why we experience our sexual feelings and memories as being so deeply personal and private. Perhaps this is why we carry them in our hearts with such care and protectiveness.

The willingness to spend time reflecting on our psychosexual story is itself an act of courage and openness. Entering into this process of reflection has its risks. Some of our memories will be warm and comforting, exciting and reassuring, perhaps even wrapped in reverie and nostalgia. But there are other memories that will bring back the searing pain of rejection, failure, or betrayal. We will likely have to confront our unfinished growth, our unresolved pain, our unnamed fears, and our lingering feelings of guilt.

Even more important than courage and honesty, therefore, is a stance of *reverence*, a willingness to be gentle with our past experience and our present selves. When we reflect on our psychosexual story, we are journeying into a paradoxical land of hope and hurt, strength and need, generosity and selfishness, love and brokenness. We are walking not only on the intense ground of ecstasy, but also on the fragile soil of unfulfilled dreams and aching memories. Most importantly, we are standing on the "holy ground" where God has laid plans for love. We want to suggest a simple guideline for approaching our psychosexual stories: Listen to your story with openness and honesty. But *do not judge* your story. Do not put unwarranted negative labels on your past, or you will "bruise" it. If it is subjected to harsh judgments, it will not be able to reveal itself as a journey with God.

Listening to Our Psychosexual Story with Trust

Our story may not be as traumatic as Celie's, but it is no less important or significant. Our understanding may not be as colorful as Shug's, but we can nevertheless trust the wisdom of our hearts. Each of our stories is a graced venture into the unknown, a sometimes painful, sometimes joyful encounter with the energies of love and hatred, acceptance and rejection, trust and betrayal. Our psychosexual story is one of the ways we discover "some of the best stuff God did."

What does it mean to listen to our psychosexual story? What does this look like in practice? How can we retrieve our memories and begin to see them as part of a journey toward integration?

Listening comes in a variety of intensities. But before it is a focused awareness, it is first an attitude of the heart — a willingness to be *receptive to the truth*. Listening is a stance of openness toward our lives and our experience. In this case, it is an openness to our sexual memories and the events and relationships that have shaped our search for love.

It is no accident that the *Shemah Israel* — the great commandment of love, which every Jewish person was to "keep in their hearts" (Dt 6:4–6) — begins with a single, dramatic command: *Listen!* Love begins and ends with listening. So too does the understanding and healing of our relational memories. Our growth and integration involve our willingness to circle back to that attentive stance.

In addition to the attitude of nonjudgmental reverence, which we mentioned above, we also recommend that people begin listening to their psychosexual stories in a stance of *prayerfulness*. Our lives are mysteries that ultimately evade our attempts to categorize them. We discover that our origin and our destiny is a love beyond our comprehension. In some way, each of us can claim the words of Jesus as our own: "I came from God and have come into the world. Now I am leaving the world and am going to God" (Jn 16:28). Living and loving is what we do between coming from God and returning to God. The most fruitful way to gain access to our story is in the presence of the God who is our beginning and our end.

In practice, listening to our psychosexual story means taking the time to be with our memories. Initially, this will probably mean time alone, time to be quiet and to let the silence speak to us, time to let memories begin to surface and play around the edges of our consciousness, time to go for walks or light a candle and just sit, time to spend jotting down memories, journaling our feelings, or, if we are so inclined, sketching images from our past.

We meet many people who report that they have few, if any, recollections of sexual feelings or experiences as children. They are often surprised to discover that once they become receptive and welcoming, the images and memories begin to return to their awareness.

Listening to our psychosexual story also involves taking the risk of asking questions. It means talking to our parents about their relationship and their memories surrounding our birth and infancy. It involves the willingness to explore our family's attitudes and messages around sexuality. It could mean conversations with our brothers and sisters or our other relatives about our shared past and early life experience.

At some point, we might also find it helpful to write out our psychosexual story for ourselves and share it with our spouse, a close friend, a spiritual director, or a counselor. When we facilitate retreats on the topic of human sexuality, we often invite participants to begin sharing their stories, at the level at which they are comfortable, in a small group setting. Listening to our personal story and sharing it with people whom we can trust can be a powerful experience of growth and healing. In various places in the text, we have interspersed reflective questions or exercises. These can be used as a starting point for listening to and exploring our psychosexual stories.

Naming Our Messages

Like Celie and Shug, our attitudes toward our sexuality are formed and shaped by the experiences, events, and people in our lives. Our earliest encounters with sexual energy — the ways that we are held, nursed, or bathed as infants, perhaps our early experiments with self-pleasuring as children — all of these can have a lasting impact on how we feel about our bodies and our sexual selves. These early experiences are not just physical stirrings or biological responses; they are emotional events that become deeply encoded in our consciousness. They are accompanied by built-in interpretations, arising from our own spontaneous discovery or from the psychic stance of our caretakers. Thus these experiences function as early sources of celebrating or shaming, valuing or humiliating, affirming or negating.

These early bodily experiences, together with their emotional "envelopes," help create our first "worldview" — our set of unspoken assumptions and expectations regarding living and loving. Most of us come into childhood and adolescence with our own implied, usually unarticulated, version of "the

birds and the bees." For many of us, these youthful attitudes
become explicit only when we enter into relationships with
persons whose background and value systems are different
from our own. Whether or not we are fully conscious of it,
we each carry deep, interiorized messages about the meaning
and mystery of sexuality.

One of the most important steps toward psychosexual integration is our ability to *name* these messages. It is our
beachhead into self-knowledge, our first initiative into reverencing our own truth. Naming our messages is just another
word for coming to know our psychosexual story.

These articulated assumptions about sexuality are part of
a wider circle of meaning that we might refer to as "core life
messages." At a surprisingly early age, when our emotional
and psychic "antenna" are extra sensitive, we tune in and internalize these messages from our parents, our caretakers, and
our family of origin. We inherit them from our classmates,
teachers, and other authority figures.

Some of these core messages are clear and verbally explicit.
For instance, on the negative side we might remember that our
parents frequently told us that we were "stupid" or that we
would "never amount to anything." Others are not necessarily
verbally stated, but are even more significant because of their
experiential impact. For example, like Celie, we might have
been physically and sexually abused. This truth may or may
not have been accompanied by words, but the outcome cries
out for recognition. It is a message that is burned forever into
our body and seared into our wounded emotions.

If we were fortunate enough to come from a reasonably healthy family, we would have inherited some affirming
messages of love and acceptance. We would still carry those
internalized affirmations today as part of our sense of personal
worth. We might remember the numerous times that our parents or caretakers spoke encouraging words to us, even when
we were naughty or crabby. We might remember the count-
less times they told us they loved us and praised our efforts
to learn.

It is not only our parents and caretakers who give us messages. We are also profoundly influenced in our attitudes
and feelings about sexuality by our culture and our peers.

In particular, the impact of our religious heritage cannot be overestimated.

When we lead weekend retreats on intimacy and human relationships, we usually invite the participants to spend time recalling and naming some of the messages that they have internalized around sexuality. We typically hear responses such as the following:

- "Our family just didn't talk about sex. The message was that the topic is taboo — which is, of course a significant message. . . . "

- "The church gave me mixed messages about sexuality. It felt like they were saying: sex is dirty; save it for somebody you love."

- "My parents were loving people, but they didn't show affection toward each other or toward us. I couldn't imagine them having sexual intercourse."

- "Each time I went on a date, my mother reminded me that the girl has to be in control; boys just can't help themselves. I got the message that boys were sexual and girls weren't."

- "In the eighth grade, the pastor took the boys to one room and Sister took the girls to another to give us the 'sex talk.' It was a pretty grim approach to sexuality. It made it seem like a secret that wasn't nice enough to talk about in mixed company."

In the past couple of decades, there are signs that the Catholic church and other Christian denominations are taking more positive steps to reaffirm the goodness of human sexuality. As the above sampling of messages reveals, this has not always been the case. Our religious traditions have not consistently given us the impression that sexuality is, in Shug's words, "some of the best stuff God did." Many of us would be at least mildly surprised to learn that "God don't think it dirty," or that "God loves them feelings best of all."

Our ability to name the messages that we have inherited from our family background and our religious heritage is an important step toward psychosexual integration. It helps us to know our inner truth and gives us the tools to begin reinterpreting these messages in a reflective and intentional way.

Reinterpreting Our Sexual Messages

In Celie's life there was a painful cycle of abuse, trauma, and oppression. But inside Celie, somewhere deep in her heart, there was also an inborn drive to seek life and healing. This energy for health was even more powerful than the personal forces of destruction that had held sway over her life for so long.

Each of us is born with this instinct for life, this yearning to become whole. However fragile and vulnerable human beings are, they also have an amazing resiliency. Our bodies have the inborn capacity to respond to physical trauma. After a wound, they immediately respond with blood coagulants that stop the bleeding. They fight infections and stabilize the shock to our system. Eventually our bodies form a protective scab, which in turn becomes a scar. Our scars are in some way "badges of courage" — symbols of our body's strength and endurance.

This striving for health is operative in our inner lives. Our minds can begin to reinterpret the meaning of life from new sources of information and insight. Our psyche can break through our illusions and denials, our self-destructive patterns of thinking, and find more creative alternatives. Our emotions, even if they are frayed and damaged, can be tended and reassured. The negative or shame-based perspective on our sexuality can be gradually replaced with a more life-affirming stance. Our sexual traumas and failures can, over the long haul, find some level of healing.

This journey toward healing and wholeness is not an easy one. It does not happen without conscious intent and a great deal of personal effort.

Nor does it happen alone. Perhaps the most striking part of Celie's challenge to reimage or reinterpret herself and her life is the role that Shug plays as friend and mentor. Shug is the companion who invites Celie to face her story, to name its pain, to acknowledge the messages that shaped her life. None of us can change our past, but we can find ways of healing it and growing from it. We cannot undo the events of our lives, but we can begin to reimage the meaning and power we give to them. In Alice Walker's novel, Shug helps Celie begin this process of rediscovery and recovery. In addition to being friend and mentor, she is also a gentle, sometimes playful confronter. She challenges Celie to reinterpret her experience, to re-examine her assumptions and expectations, and then to decide how she wants to reshape her future.

Shug is a metaphor for those who come into our lives as healing mentors and friends. These people are unexpected gifts, reminders of God's unconditional love in the midst of life. Who are the Shugs in our lives? Who are the friends, the teachers, the colleagues, the counselors, the beloved, who have helped us name our history, and then invited us to healing and new vision?

Whoever they are, God has given them to us as part of a loving plan. A plan for our welfare and not for harm. A plan for our relational wholeness. A plan to give us a future with hope.

QUESTIONS FOR REFLECTION AND SHARING

These questions have been designed to help you personalize what you have just read. They are a way of getting in touch with your own story, of exploring what in you needs further growth or healing. Do not feel that you have to respond to all of them. Also, you may wish to reflect on them over several occasions. You may find it helpful to spend some time in prayer with them, to record your responses in your journal, or in some cases to share your responses with a close friend or significant other.

1. Have you experienced times of "emotional exile" in your life? Try to recall the persons and events that surrounded those feelings. If the emotions that surface tell you that something is unfinished or in need of healing, spend some time in journaling and/or prayer. You might also consider confiding these memories to a close friend, spouse, counselor, or spiritual director.

2. Ira Progroff developed a journaling device that he called "Stepping Stones" — a way of outlining the major turning points or transition experiences in our life stories. What are the "stepping stones" in your psychosexual story? Try to make a list of seven or eight of the most significant events or formative relationships in your life story. What do these turning points reveal about your search for love and intimacy?

3. What were the "core life messages" during your growing up years? More specifically, what were the messages — verbal or nonverbal — about sexuality in your family? Perhaps you might want to spend some time discussing this with members of your family.

4. Who are the "Shugs" in your life? The friends, teachers, or mentors who helped you come to a more affirming understanding of sexuality and intimacy? Have you ever told them how much they meant in your life?

5. What would you like to reimage or reinterpret in your attitudes and inherited messages toward sexuality? Jot down some of your reflections. Bring them to prayer or share them with someone you trust.

3

PATHWAY TO LOVE

An Overview of Psychosexual Development

I have come that they may have life, and have it to the full.

— John 10:10

This declaration by Jesus in the fourth gospel serves as a "mission statement" for Christian living. It reminds us that we are created for an expansive purpose — to enter into our human experience and to discover there a *fullness*, a wellspring of relationships, feelings, and creativity. It tells us that God has more in mind for us than just "staying out of trouble." We are created to become whole persons, not just moral robots. We are called to embrace life, not to avoid it, to welcome its energy and to pursue its possibilities.

The Greek word that the author of John uses for "life" is *zoe*, a term that implies a *dynamic wholeness*. It is more comprehensive and integral than *bios* (referring to the conduct of everyday living, with its ambitions and possessions) or *psyche* (life, or the soul as the organizing principle). *Zoe* encompasses the physical and relational energy of our selfhood; it implies both earthiness and transcendence, the now and the not-yet, our immediate needs and our eternal hungers.

Our sexuality and the quest for human intimacy are an integral part of this dynamic wholeness. In the gospel vision, love — both human and divine — is the central way in which

35

zoe is revealed and expressed. Similarly, psychosexual development is the growth process through which our capacity to love comes to fruition. It is the presence of "cosmic allurement" in our flesh, the other-orienting energy of God in our lives.

In this chapter we will outline what we mean by psychosexual development. At the outset, we want to make it clear that we are approaching it not just as a behavioral process, but as a pathway to love. Psychosexual development is another word for our journey toward life — *life to the full*.

The notion of "development" is not new to the behavioral sciences or to contemporary spirituality. During the twentieth century, our understanding of human life has moved from a static perspective to an evolutionary one. Most of us no longer think of maturity as an event that takes place in our early adult years. Today we speak of human maturation in terms of life stages, life cycles, and life tasks. We understand it as an ongoing process involving all aspects of our lives and relationships.

This evolving vision of human growth has touched almost every aspect of human behavior. Jean Piaget and others have pioneered studies around *cognitive* development. Other researchers have studied *social* and *psychological* development. Erik Erikson gave us the "eight stages of life" and their corresponding tasks. Daniel Levinson and Gail Sheehey explored the implications of the adult life cycle. Lawrence Kohlberg and Carol Gilligan have written about *moral* development, and James Fowler speaks of the stages of *faith* development.

More recently, this understanding of ongoing maturation has also begun to influence the way we understand our sexuality and our capacity to enter into and sustain human relationships. New research has given us expanded data regarding the manner in which human persons grow sexually and relationally.

In the past few decades there are signs that the Catholic church is also entering into serious dialogue with the behavioral sciences around the topic of sexuality. This conversation includes an emerging awareness in the church's teaching of the reality of psychosexual development. In 1975, the Vatican promulgated its "Declaration on Certain Questions Concerning Sexual Ethics." The document begins with this statement:

According to contemporary scientific research, the human person is so profoundly affected by sexuality that it must be considered as one of the factors which give to each individual's life the principle traits that distinguish it. In fact it is from sex that the human person receives the characteristics which, on the biological, psychological and spiritual levels, make that person a man or a woman, *and thereby largely condition his or her progress towards maturity and insertion into society* [emphasis ours].[7]

Although the ideas contained in this passage are expressed in rather abstract language, it is nevertheless clear that the Vatican is approaching human sexuality from a *developmental*, rather than a static point of view.

Why does sexuality so "profoundly affect" our personhood? What are the characteristics that condition our "progress toward maturity and insertion into society"? These are precisely the issues that we are addressing here.

A similar emphasis on the developmental aspects of our sexuality is contained in the 1991 document published by the United States Catholic Conference, *Human Sexuality: A Catholic Perspective for Education and Lifelong Learning*. This helpful instruction provides a positive image of human sexuality as a gift from God. It places psychosexual growth in the context of our call to "wholeness and holiness," and concludes with a suggested framework for ongoing education in human sexuality.[8]

What Is Psychosexual Development?

What do we mean when we use the term "psychosexual development?" What does it imply regarding the relationship between our "psyche" and our sexual energy?

Psychosexual development is another word for "growing up" in our relational lives. It is our personal journey toward integration as embodied human persons. Psychosexual development refers to that dynamic interplay of experiences, circumstances, phases, tasks, awarenesses, and decisions that lead us toward mature and loving relationships. It is a process of growth that embraces all aspects of our human reality.

More specifically, we can speak of healthy psychosexual development as including the following six dimensions:

- *physical:* The genetic, biological, hormonal factors that influence our sexual response from the first moments of conception and throughout the seasons of our lives.

- *cognitive:* Accurate and adequate sexual knowledge; the positive perception of our bodies; beliefs that reverence self and others.

- *emotional:* Being "at home" with our body; being aware of and comfortable with our sexual feelings; having healthy feelings toward others.

- *social:* Relating to others in unself-conscious ways; having the capacity for self-disclosure; being able to sustain friendship and intimacy.

- *moral:* Valuing the attitudes and actions that are necessary for ongoing sexual integration; expressions of our sexuality that are faithful, healthy, and other-enriching; behaviors that are congruent with our life commitments.

- *spiritual:* Affirming the presence of God and the sacred in our sexual feelings and expressions; coming to recognize that sexuality and spirituality are not enemies, but friends.

When any of these six dimensions are absent or limited, or if they develop in unhealthy ways, our journey toward sexual integration will in some way be hindered or slowed down, perhaps even halted altogether. As a result, our sexual energy will likely be expressed in ways that are hurtful to ourselves or others. Some of these unhealthy attitudes or harmful behaviors include the following:

- The inability to make accurate assessments of potentially dangerous sexual behavior in ourselves or others.

- Discomfort with ourselves socially, physically, and emotionally.

- The inability to develop and sustain relationships that give life; coldness and distance in relating to people.

- A tendency to be excessively judgmental or self-righteous in our attitudes toward the sexual behavior of others.

- The inability to be faithful to primary commitments and relationships.

- Involvement in sexually unhealthy or abusive behaviors, for example, casual or anonymous sex, use of pornography, deriving sexual gratification from children, the compartmentalization of one's sexuality.

In the past few decades there has been widespread interest in "stage" theories of human development. These theories propose that we must pass through *predictable stages* that are characterized by *particular tasks* that must be accomplished at each stage. An essential aspect of this approach is that we cannot move on to the next stage until the tasks of the previous one have been successfully completed.

These theories have been useful in helping us understand the underlying direction of human growth, as well as the particular challenges at any one phase of our life journey.

More recently, however, the stage theories of development have come under criticism for what some consider to be their proclivity to oversimplify the complex dynamism of human growth. They have also been challenged for their tendency to categorize or compartmentalize our behavior in an overly facile way.

Models of Psychosexual Development

"Love is a many splendored thing." These words from a popular song remind us of the multifaceted nature of human relationships and sexuality. Love is not only a many splendored thing; it is an elusive, confusing, and often painful reality. It can be as fragile as a flower or as powerful as a raging tide, as fleeting as the passing seasons or as eternal as the stars. In the end our words fail us and our hearts fall silent. In one way or another, love will always be a mystery beyond our grasp, if not beyond our reach.

As we begin outlining the stages of psychosexual development, it might be good to remind ourselves of this fundamental truth. Our human experience is ultimately a mystery that lies outside the limits of science and beyond our ability to comprehend it, let alone adequately describe it. There is no philosophical system or theological treatise that can fully explain our yearning for love.

It is not our intention, therefore, to summarize our reality as sexual persons in a schema or limit it to a series of developmental stages. Just as photographs are only momentary glimpses or passing hints of real life, so too are attempts to develop various models of psychosexual development. We humans grope toward the truth by using stories, metaphors, and parables. We dance around our experience with similes and analogies. And, in the words of the medieval philosophers, "Every analogy limps." It is precisely through analogy and metaphor that we give shape and form to our learning. If we respect the analogical limitations, we can also honor their legitimate insights. In this case, perhaps we can think of human sexuality as the terrain — the holy ground — that we are exploring. The schematic models and developmental stages are initial attempts to describe that terrain. They are "life maps" for our sexual geography. They function as "sightings" on the psyche's horizon, as trailmarkers along the pathway of human growth.

We are proposing two models or schemas of psychosexual development that will serve as a context for the chapters that follow.

Model I. The first (see Figure 1) is based on a "stage" approach to human growth. It is a more linear and clearly defined pattern of development. It also has the advantage of chronicling our growth according to the built-in category of age. Among its disadvantages are the tendencies that we mentioned above, namely, the danger of oversimplifying the tasks of a particular time and the tendency to compartmentalize our experience.[9]

Model II. The second model (Figure 2) is more circular and convergent. It recognizes that our growth unfolds as much in cycles as it does in stages and that we cannot always point to neatly delineated transition times from one stage to another. It also suggests that we usually do not accomplish all the tasks for any one phase of our lives. More than likely, we will have

Figure 1
STAGES OF PSYCHOSEXUAL DEVELOPMENT

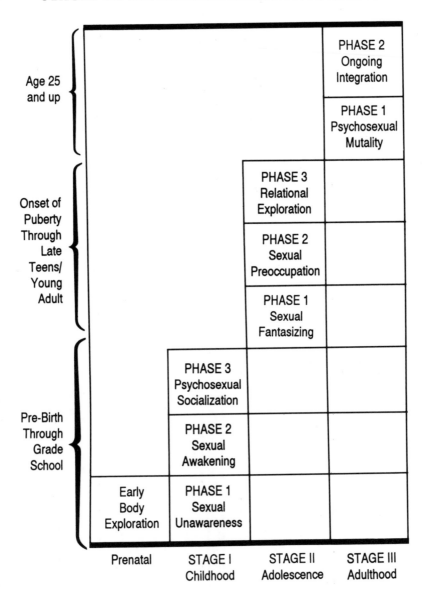

Figure 2
CYCLES OF PSYCHOSEXUAL DEVELOPMENT

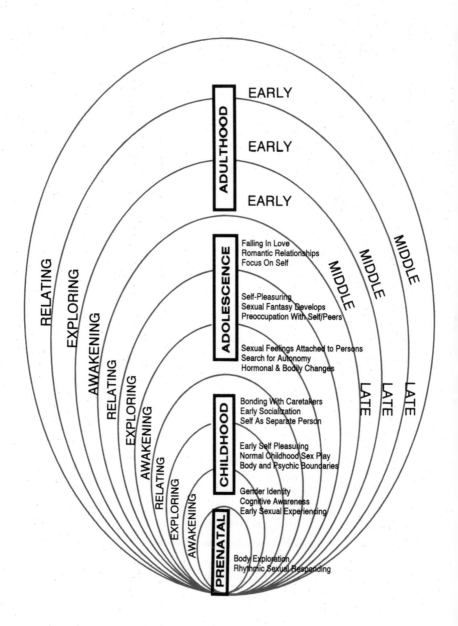

to "circle back" and attend to the "unfinished business" in our path toward integration.

In this second model, there is room for the stages of development to overlap and intermingle. It acknowledges that there are several stages of "sexual awakening," many cycles of "exploring," and multiple phases of "relating" in our lives.

In the chapters that follow we will be combining both of these models of development. For the sake of clarity and logical progression, we are employing the first model for the sequence of topics. Thus, we will address four stages of psychosexual development: *prenatal, childhood, adolescence*, and *adulthood*.

At the same time, we will attempt to integrate the wisdom of the second model by reflecting on the recurring cycles of growth that move us toward relational maturity. The fundamental rhythms of *awakening, exploring*, and *relating* unfold and then recur. Thus, as we move through the seasons of our lives, we address some of the same fundamental tasks in a more conscious, intentional, and responsible manner.

The Underlying Direction of Psychosexual Development

There are several important questions that this initial overview of psychosexual development raises for our daily living. What practical information can we learn here for ourselves and the formation of our children? How can our knowledge of these stages help us to love more fully and deeply? What do they tell us about the relationship between human wholeness and Christian holiness? What is the underlying trajectory — the fundamental direction of our development?

These are questions that will be addressed more in depth in this book. However, even at this early stage of reflection, there are some initial conclusions that we can make regarding the basic dynamism of our growth toward psychosexual integration. From our earliest stirrings in the womb and throughout the cycles of our lives, there are four qualities that underlie healthy human and sexual development. These four ongoing "marks of health" are (1) emerging self-awareness, (2) responsible freedom, (3) developing creativity, and (4) deepening capacity for intimacy.

Emerging Self-Awareness

Being a human person implies the ability to say "I am." It is the unique way that each of us images and participates in the divine "I AM" of God. Even before we can say the word "I," there is already an experiential center, a spontaneous source of awakening, exploring, and relating in our lives. This primal awareness gradually emerges into the sense of being a separate self — different from our parents or primary caretakers; part of, but not the same as, our environment.

Self-awareness continues to unfold through our early experiences of bodily exploration and gender identity. It develops further during the time of youthful socialization, when we begin to feel "self-conscious" and desirous of more privacy. It flowers in adolescence as we struggle with dependency and autonomy on our road to claiming our individuality. If we are healthy, self-awareness will continue to deepen throughout our adult years. This knowledge of being a separate, conscious center of embodied life is essential to our lives as lovers and friends.

Responsible Freedom

As human infants, we are dependent on our caretakers in more ways and for a longer time than most other animal species. Our ability to be independent — to "stand on our own" physically and then emotionally — comes relatively slowly. But when it begins to happen, we reach out eagerly to claim it. The innate drive to choose our own way — to decide our relationships, our values, our career, and the manner in which we express our sexual energy — is one of the most distinctive marks of being human.

Before the emergence of self-consciousness, our freedom is primarily expressed as *spontaneity* of movement and physical response. As infants, we do not consciously direct the inborn rhythms of our sexual energy, but we do respond to these physical stirrings with a spirit of play and enjoyment. A little later, as two-year-olds, the response of freedom becomes the resolute "No!" — the first indicator that we are aware of our ability to direct and shape our lives. As adolescents, the tasks of freedom are contoured around our search for autonomy and a desire to "be on our own."

From our earliest years we begin to learn that freedom is not just spontaneity; it is also *responsibility* for the implications of our decisions. It is the willingness to carry the consequences of our choices. In the area of psychosexual development, this growing sense of accountability is revealed in an important psychic transition: the gradual shift from experiencing our sexuality as a "cosmic energy" toward understanding it as a personal gift and responsibility. It also implies that we follow an ethical vision in the ways that we choose to express our sexuality.

Developing Creativity

When self-awareness and freedom converge, the human outcome is *creativity* — the capacity for renewing and reshaping creation, the ability to participate in making new life. It is unfortunate that we tend to reduce sexual creativity to procreation — the biological capacity to produce offspring. This physical "begetting" is the most obvious form of human creativity, but it is not the only way that we bring about new life.

Long before we reach the age of puberty, sexual creativity is taking place in our lives. To confirm this we need only reflect on the rhythms of sexual response that begin *in utero* and that continue in some form throughout our lives. When we are young we also experiment with communication, invent words, give birth to dreams, nurture feelings, and create fantasies. As we grow into adulthood, our lives become productive through our work and in the ways that we help build a more just and peaceful world.

Our creativity can deepen still further to become *generativity*, a life-enhancing quality that flows, not just from our procreative desire or our productive efforts, but from our inner being as human persons.

Deepening Capacity for Intimacy

The ability to relate — to connect physically, emotionally, and spiritually — begins at the earliest moments of our lives. As infants, it takes the form of a primordial "bonding" between the child and mother or primary caretaker. As preschoolers, it is the slow emergence of ego-identity and the desire to be close to our playmates, siblings, grandparents, aunts and uncles, and our family pet. In grade school it is the discovery of "best friends" or membership on a team.

In early adolescence we begin to experience romantic feelings. Perhaps we fall in love for the first time. If we continue to grow in healthy self-confidence, our adult lives will be marked by a deepening hunger and a corresponding capacity to share more mutually and honestly with those whom we choose as life companions.

From the point of view of psychology, we can describe *intimacy as loving behavior that is manifested through self-disclosure*. The gift of mutual sharing between two adults as partners and friends is, in one sense, the fullest flowering of our sexual energy. It is a gift that can never be fully realized, a well that will not run dry, a mystery that will lead us into deeper closeness with God.

Wholeness and Holiness

How do these four qualities reflect the relationship between human growth and the life of grace? Perhaps we can best answer this by asking a further question. From the perspective of psychological health, how do we describe someone who is reasonably self-aware, responsibly free, creative, and able to share authentic intimacy? Do we not say that this person is *mature*? By maturity, we clearly mean more than just being physically "grown up." We are referring to a certain balance, an integration of gifts, a capacity to relate to others, a *wholeness* of life.

From the perspective of Christian life, how do we describe someone with the same or similar characteristics, viewed now in the light of faith and weighed in the balance of love? Would we not say that this person is *holy*? And by holiness we are referring to something more than just keeping moral rules or engaging in pious practices. We are speaking of the same kind of balance and integration of gifts, the same capacity to relate to others with commitment and love.

In other words, holiness is simply human wholeness from the perspective of grace. The Latin language retains this fundamental identity of our human lives and our graced existence in God. In the Vulgate translation of the Bible, the Latin word *salus* means both salvation and health, holiness and wholeness.

Chastity: Journey Toward Relational Wholeness

In our culture — and to some extent also in our churches — the virtue of chastity does not have a very positive image. Most people tend to think of it in rather negative terms — usually as a list of "don'ts" and "shouldn'ts" in relationship to sexual experience.

Obviously, there is a place for ethical guidelines in the area of sexuality. Chastity *is* morally demanding. It calls us to a disciplined way of life based on reverence in relationships and wholehearted love of God. Whether we are a married couple, a single person, or a vowed celibate, chastity challenges us to respect the powerful and sometimes chaotic energy of sexuality in our lives.[10]

But in our contemporary society, there is also a need for a more affirming approach to chastity. We are attempting to develop an experiential basis for such an approach in this book. In one sense, chastity is a way of talking about psychosexual integration in the light of gospel values. It is the graced pattern of growth and commitment that leads us to life — life to the full. Approaching psychosexual development in this way can also help us to understand the "intrinsic ethic" of sexuality — the inner trajectory of growth that leads us both to human wholeness *and* Christian holiness.

We can't assume that, just because we have bodies, we are *incarnate*. Incarnation is more than a condition; it is a journey, a process of embracing our embodied lives. There are many people who seek to escape from their bodiliness by denying or repressing their sexual energy. There are others who seek to leap out of the human condition by engaging in compulsive or addictive sexual behaviors that are harmful to themselves and others. Chastity — the movement toward psychosexual integration — involves the long and arduous journey of *becoming incarnate*, of entering reverently and responsibly into our flesh, so that our sexual energy becomes a vehicle for love rather than selfishness. Chastity is "life to the full" in our psychosexual lives.

QUESTIONS FOR REFLECTION AND SHARING

These questions have been designed to help you personalize what you have just read. They are a way of getting in touch with your own story, of exploring what in you needs further growth or healing. Do not feel that you have to respond to all of them. Also, you may wish to reflect on them over several occasions. You may find it helpful to spend some time in prayer with them, to record your responses in your journal, or in some cases to share your responses with a close friend or significant other.

1. Which of the models of psychosexual development (see Figures 1 and 2) do you find most helpful in understanding your personal growth? Can you identify times of awakening, exploring, and relating in your life story?

2. Spend some time reflecting on the four basic characteristics in the "growth trajectory" of psychosexual development, namely, emerging self-awareness, responsible freedom, developing creativity, and deepening capacity for intimacy.

3. In what ways have you become more "self-aware" in your adult years?

4. What have been the breakdowns and/or breakthroughs for you in the area of responsibility and freedom, especially as this relates to sexuality and interpersonal relationships?

5. How are you a *creative* person in your life and relationships?

6. Has your capacity to be more self-disclosive — more intimate with those closest to you — grown or deepened? How? Where do you see signs of this growth?

7. Take some time to reflect on and, if possible, put in writing what *chastity* means to you. Share some of your thoughts with your loved ones or your children.

4

KNIT TOGETHER
IN MY MOTHER'S WOMB

Psychosexual Development and Prenatal Life

You created my inmost self,
knit me together in my mother's womb.
For so many marvels I thank you;
a wonder am I, and all your works are wonders.

— Psalm 139:13–14

The psalmist gives testimony to the familiar Judeo-Christian belief that God has been involved in each of our lives from the beginning. A very personal God shapes our inmost self, knits us together, fashions us into a wonder amid all the other wonders of creation. The psalmist offers an image of God that is as earthy and homespun as it is divine: God is a worker of yarn, one who knits each of us together with the same precision and care that goes into the creation of a fine wool garment. Like the slow, methodical work of the knitter, God threads and weaves and loops each strand of potential humanity into a unique person. And, like the finished wool garment, by the time we are ready for birth, each fiber of our being has passed through the hands of a knitting God.

Prenatal Sexual Development

Through the advances of medical science, we have come to know a great deal more about the specifics of being "knit together" in the womb. Things that the psalmist took on faith we can watch on an ultrasound screen. We know that our journey from a single microscopic cell (the fertilized egg) to a fully developed body involves complex cellular and hormonal interactions that resemble slow, purposeful knitting. Tenderly and quietly, we are woven into a being that is truly a wonder!

The process of psychosexual development involves a long journey. We have been traveling from the beginning. Soon after our conception, we made our way to our mother's uterine wall, and began to nestle into our first growing place. At that time, we were only a microscopic ball of cells.

Then a series of rapid transformations began to take place. The inner part of our embryonic selves differentiated into two layers, the endoderm and the ectoderm. Next, a third layer, the mesoderm, formed between them. It was from this center layer of cells that our reproductive and circulatory systems eventually evolved. Sexuality and the heart — they were together from the beginning.

From the perspective of embryology, sexuality, as symbolized by our reproductive system, lives at the core of our lives. It lies between the layers of the inner and outer worlds of our humanity, touching and influencing both of them. It is possible to consider this simply an evolutionary coincidence or a developmental necessity, having no symbolic meaning. Indeed, this is how many in the scientific community might regard it. However, our approach in this book is not merely to report the results of scientific research regarding prenatal development. Rather, it is to observe the data and look for its deeper meaning. It is to acknowledge the knitter.

Perhaps it is not by accident that our reproductive and circulatory systems come from the same layer of tissue. It is as though the designer of humanity intended that our sexuality and our hearts ought to be connected in some primordial way. They ought to lie near each other, to unfold together, to be a flesh-and-blood symbol of the psychosexual integration to which humanity is called. Sexuality and the heart would be associated from the outset. Springing as they do from a common origin, they would know, at some deep level of being, that neither could be complete without the other.

Personalizing Our Prenatal Development

We know much more about the physiology of our prenatal psychosexual development than we do about its psychology. We can now chronicle, with almost day-to-day precision, the gradual internal and external sexual development of the tiny embryo from about the sixth week of gestation. What does it look like? What process did our own sexuality go through as it began the journey of incarnation?

As males and females, we shared a common starting place. For the first twenty-eight days following our conception, we were physiologically identical, except for our differing sex chromosomes. By the fifth or the sixth week of our gestation, the structures that would eventually develop into either male or female reproductive systems had already been formed. At this point, we had a pair of gonads, each with a potential to develop in either a male or a female direction. Our rudimentary external genitals looked identical.

Early human embryology reveals a powerful truth about our sexuality. It has been with us from the beginning. Even before it was overtly expressed, it was present to us as a quiet background energy, a silent fire.

We were knit together in our mother's wombs. There, in the wet and warm place where human life begins, our bodies were formed. Cell knit to cell. Neuron connected to neuron. One heartbeat following another. Some call it reproduction. To the psalmist, it was a wonder. For the Christian, it is incarnation once again.

The Inmost Self: The Emergence of Personality

As wondrous as our prenatal development is, there is more to it than our physical formation. The psalmist hints of it when he speaks of the "inmost self." There is something more than flesh, something of an innerness that is knit into the fabric of our being. It permeates our flesh, but is not synonymous with

it. The psalmist would not have been speaking of a soul because the concept of a "soul" as distinct from the body would
have been foreign to the Hebrew mentality. The inmost self: it
is with us from the beginning. It is that part of us that involves
our core identity, our uniqueness. Psychology might refer to
it as our personality.

The inmost self. Whatever "innerness" is there from the beginning, we know that it includes our sexuality. Perhaps more
than any other dimension of our potential humanness, our sexual identity as male or female is there from the earliest stages
of the process of conception. The united sperm and egg give
us either two x chromosomes (female, xx) or an x and a y
(male, xy), thereby giving us a sexual identity (chromosomal
gender) as among the first of the many characteristics we will
carry for the rest of our lives.

Before medical tests are able to determine if our eyes are to
be blue or gray, our hair black or red, our skeletal frame large
or small, they can identify our chromosomal gender. Before
thought is given to whether we will be bold or shy, musical
or athletic, imaginative or industrious, we are decidedly male
or female. We are physically sexual from the beginning. As
the Vatican document notes, it is from sex that we find the
starting point that will condition our lives.

The "Quickening" of Sexuality

Most of us have heard about the historic first movement that
occurs about the fifth month of our gestation. It happens when
we have enough "body mass" for our physical motion to be
perceived by our mothers. But there is another kind of "quickening" that takes place later that is less familiar. It involves an
early form of psychic awakening — the first stirring of our
"inmost selves." Somewhere between the twenty-eighth and
thirty-second weeks of gestation, our cerebral cortex becomes
mature enough to support consciousness.[11]

It begins with a perception of fragmentary sensations. Our
flesh receives messages from both inside and outside itself.
Kicking and stretching are accompanied by the interior movements of early awareness. Soon we begin reacting to the
environment in which we find ourselves. We hear voices, some

familiar, some that are strange to us. We listen to sounds. We have our first emotional responses. Slowly our new flesh begins to communicate with our "inmost selves."

During the third trimester of our gestation, we could suck our thumbs, hiccough, swallow, and produce what some specialists believe to be purposeful movements. We could experience pleasure. We could become agitated. We startled to sudden, loud sounds. Already, our preferences were forming. Characteristics were taking shape. Emotional responses were occurring daily. And woven through all of it was an exciting energy that would permeate all of our lives. It was the energy of connection. It was sexuality.

We are generally not accustomed to thinking of the soft, cuddly babies that emerge from the womb as sexual, at least not sexual beyond being male or female. But advances in medical technology and theological reflection are giving us new awareness about the existence and meaning of prenatal sexuality. Until recent years, most textbooks on human sexuality limited their descriptions of prenatal sexuality to the biological formation of genital structures. Increasingly, however, they are adding chapters that go beyond physiology to include the psychological components of our early sexual development.

What are they saying? What are we able to know about our earliest efforts to integrate our psychosexuality? How does our "quickening" stretch beyond the physical movements of our flesh and begin to write the first chapter of our psychosexual story?

Body Awareness: The Beginnings of Psychosexual Development

It has been said that the largest sexual organ of the human body is the skin and that the most important sexual organ is the brain. Studies have consistently shown that the human person needs skin touch throughout life simply to survive. Infants reared without sufficient handling either die or grow up to be socially disabled as adults. The relationship between early physical touch and later interpersonal competence is a strong one.

For each of us, the earliest and most important form of

touch was *self-touch*. It began *in utero* with our first halting, searching movements. Mouth-hand touch, hand-body touch, and body-uterine wall contact provided us with our first awareness of our incarnate selves. We didn't experience ourselves as separate from our mothers until long after birth. But our early contacts with the feel of our bodies and the sensate messages of the uterine muscle, the warm water, and the increasingly small space all contributed to what we might consider the primordial awareness of our body boundaries.

Even though we did not have the cognitive capacity to name these experiences or to form conscious memories of them before birth, our bodies will always remember. Soft places. Hard places. Places that move and places that don't. Uncomfortable experiences. Pleasurable ones. They all went into the memory bank that is stored in our flesh for all time.

What does all of this have to do with our sexuality? First, we want to emphasize that sexuality, even in its earliest stages, goes beyond genitality. Before it is a pelvic urge, it is a body awareness. We awaken to our whole physical selves before we awaken to our genital desires. Our first psychosexual task is to begin to gain a sense of body awareness. Before birth, we do this by exploring our own developing flesh. We rub. We suck. We kick. We touch everything we can reach — or everything that we discover within our reach. The more our flesh becomes familiar to us, the more we will be able to take responsibility for its desires.

Prenatal Influences and Adult Sexual Behavior

Because as adults we cannot consciously remember our prenatal experience, it can seem like a faraway, unreal part of our existence. Yet much happened during our prenatal life that still exerts its influence today: how intensely we feel our sexual energy; who we find attractive; the ways we express our maleness or femaleness.

There are many prenatal processes related to psychosexual development that scientists are exploring today. They have to do with the ways that hormones, genes, and various intrauterine conditions influence our later adult sexual interests and behaviors. Early research in this area has suggested that such things as the intensity of our adult sex drive, the strength and direction of our sexual orientation, and even the types of cues that will later evoke sexual arousal may have their origins in prenatal development.

While it is now widely accepted that such factors as prenatal hormones exert an influence on later psychosexuality, the precise degree to which they do so is unknown. Most researchers in this area agree that both prenatal hormones and postnatal nurturant experiences interact to help shape adult sexual behavior. However, they experience less agreement on the relative strength of each of these influences.

For example, some behavioral scientists believe that hormones circulating in the bloodstream of the fetus actually program brain physiology for the psychosexual interests and behaviors that will be with a person throughout life. These can be modified, perhaps, but not completely changed once brain programming has taken place. Other researchers find that prenatal hormonal programming is much more subject to postnatal social communication and learning and that the psychosexuality of the human person continues to undergo critical development in the weeks, months, and years following birth.

No doubt, the "nature/nurture" debate will continue to exist among scientists as new discoveries on both sides of the issue take place. What seems important for those of us wishing to explore the meaning of prenatal sexuality is not to place it in competition with postnatal experience. Both prenatal and postnatal events influence our lives. We know that sex hormones (androgens and estrogens) are present during gestation and that they have a direct influence on our developing sexuality. To continue to learn more about their precise action can only bring us into closer contact with the God who knit us in the womb.

As believing persons, we recognize that we are destined for love, for relationships. We also know that we are always in process, always growing, always moving toward greater levels of integration in all aspects of our lives. Whatever happens prenatally must be directed toward that end — toward the development of the capacity to love.

Unlike the sexual behavior of other species, our sexual behavior is governed by more than a mating instinct or a pelvic urge that has been irrevocably programmed into our brains. Our potential for sexual union is not regulated by cycles of fertility, nor is our desire for genital contact limited to reproductive fulfillment. Our yearning for human closeness goes far beyond that which can be satisfied by physical union alone.

In our adult lives, hormones, when functioning normally, certainly influence each of these aspects of our sexuality, but they do not exert total control over them. Unlike sheep, we are not hormonal robots. We have an "inmost self" that can make decisions, be faithful, and act responsibly. Our movement toward psychosexual integration involves all dimensions of ourselves learning to function in relationship to each other. When this is happening, our cognitive capacities inform and direct our bodily drives. Our physical passions warm our mental processes. Our feelings and our moral values communicate with each other. While we do not see a full flowering of this kind of integration until adulthood, it is already starting *in utero*. The garment of our whole selves is being woven. The knitting together has begun. It is a marvel!

The Physiological Cycles of Sexual Responding

Because medical technology enables observance of the fetus *in utero*, knowledge about the actual process of prenatal body exploration and sexual responding is increasing, especially for the third trimester. Sooner or later, babies discover their genitals and seem to experience pleasure in touching them. An increase in both heart rate and physical movement are associated with genital touch during later prenatal development.

It also appears that vaginal lubrication in the female and penile erection in the male begin to occur before birth.[12] Some neonatologists speculate that these responses may initiate a rhythmic cycle of sexual responding that is known to exist in children and to continue in adults throughout life. Although the precise schedule of such a cycle is unknown, it is known that adults experience these responses during sleep on a regular, cyclic basis.

Whatever the particular frequency and rhythm, human beings have a "built-in" sexual response that begins before we are born. We have been "knit together" that way. Our faith prompts us to regard it as a marvel of God's creative purpose.

Simply knowing of the existence of these responses, in some form, in all human persons, prompts us to ask the deeper questions that science cannot answer.

We do not need to wait for statistics and data in order to bring theological reflection into the arena of prenatal sexuality. Dialogue between religion and science must be an ongoing part of our search for truth. Pope John Paul II emphasized the importance of such dialogue. In 1989, in an address marking the anniversary of the publication of Newton's *Principia Mathematica*, John Paul II had this to say:

> Science can purify religion from error and superstition; religion can purify science from idolatry and false absolutes. The unprecedented opportunity we have today is for a common interactive relationship in which each discipline retains its integrity and yet is radically open to the discoveries and insights of the other.[13]

Previous papal leaders have made similar statements about the value of science. Pope Pius XII stressed the importance of allowing the truth of scientific discoveries to rest not on the religious beliefs of scientists, but on the correspondence of their findings to reality:

> The observations of Hippocrates which have been recognized as exact, the discoveries of Pasteur, or Mendel's laws of heredity, do not owe the truth of their content to the moral and religious ideas of their authors. They are not "pagan" because Hippocrates was pagan nor are they Christian because Pasteur and Mendel were Christians. These scientific achievements are true for the reason and to the extent that they correspond with reality.[14]

Prenatal Sexuality and Theology

Our capacity to respond sexually begins before we are born. The all-permeating energy of sexuality that fills every cell in our bodies is knit into us from the beginning. It intensifies as we grow. As soon as our hands are able to engage in reaching, touching movements, we find our noses, our mouths, our toes, our genitals, and begin the wondrous journey of self-discovery. Our first tentative touches tell us something about the God who chose sexuality as the vehicle of humanity's differentiation and made it more than a reproductive capacity.

God chose sexuality. God invested sexuality with fire, with energy, with passion and put it in our bodies. Why would God do such a thing? Could not the all-knowing God have designed something less volatile to ensure the reproduction of the human species? Would not our creator be capable of thinking of a mating plan that would function only during those times when conception was needed or desired, thus avoiding unnecessary sexual passion? At the very least, if God did see a need for some occasional sexual desire in human beings, why introduce it into the bodies of babies? If it has purpose only in marriage, why is its energy being experienced by healthy infants?

It seems that we have two choices: We can either assume, as did Augustine, that God did not intend to create sexual passion at all and that somehow it "slipped in" apart from God's plan. Or, conversely, we can believe that human sexuality is the purposefully designed intention of a creative God. This is a God who "thought up" pelvic pleasure, orgasm, and sexual passion and placed a capacity for these experiences into our bodies, into our "inmost selves," from the very beginning.

Perhaps God sensed in advance that human beings would be fearful and suspicious of such a powerful energy and begin to find ways to blunt or deny it rather than embrace it and carry it responsibly. Perhaps that is why it is knit into us so early. The rhythmic cycles of sexual responding stand as beacons to us, constant reminders to us that we are sexual. Already *in utero*, our sexual responses are as close as our heartbeat, as steady as our growth. Our early explorations of our bodies are our first sexual acts. Our discoveries of pleasurable sensations are our first sexual teachers. Through them we learn that flesh is good, that touch is associated with comfort. Most importantly, we gain the first rudimentary awarenesses that our flesh belongs to us. We are in charge of it. It is ours. We are the first to touch it, the first to feel its contours, the first to produce its wondrous variety of sensations. There, in the quiet recesses of the womb, where no one has yet taught us otherwise, we experience our flesh as entirely safe and fully worthy of our caress. And so we suck and lick and touch. We receive our body's gift of pleasures. The knitter is pleased.

QUESTIONS FOR REFLECTION AND SHARING

These questions have been designed to help you personalize what you have just read. They are a way of getting in touch with your own story, of exploring what in you needs further growth or healing. Do not feel that you have to respond to all of them. Also, you may wish to reflect on them over several occasions. You may find it helpful to spend some time in prayer with them, to record your responses in your journal, or in some cases to share your responses with a close friend or significant other.

1. What do you know about the circumstances of your mother's pregnancy while she carried you? How was her physical and emotional health? Did she smoke, drink alcohol, or use any drugs while pregnant? How long had it been since she delivered a previous child before she became pregnant with you? What kind of support system did she have?

2. How did your mother spend her days while she was pregnant with you? What was the level of emotional stability in her environment at the time? Who else lived in the house? What would it have been like to be a baby in her womb?

3. What do you know about your mother's labor and delivery with you? Where were you born? Who attended your birth? Were there any complications? Did you ever hear your birth story?

4. What questions do you have about your own prenatal experience?

5. How do you think you have been affected by your prenatal experiences? Do you recognize any connection between: Your mother's pregnancy experiences and your current level of self-esteem? Sense of belonging? Degree of interior calmness or anxiety? Right to be here?

5

LET THE CHILDREN COME TO ME

Psychosexual Development During Childhood

> Now they were bringing even infants to him that he might touch them; and when the disciples saw it, they rebuked them. But Jesus called them to him, saying, "Let the children come to me, and do not hinder them; for to such belongs the kingdom of God."
>
> — Luke 18:15–16

The people brought infants. The Greek word used to describe the infants indicates that they were newborns still at the breast. The parents wanted only one thing — that Jesus *touch* their tiny babies.

This scene is often referred to as "the blessing of the children." While Mark and Matthew portray Jesus laying his hands on the children and blessing them, Luke omits any suggestion of formal benediction. The Greek word, *hapto*, means "to touch" or "to hold." For Luke, it was enough to present Jesus simply *touching* the infants. The people in Luke's story wanted Jesus to extend to their babies the kind of affirmation that comes from human touch. They had heard of the rabbi whose hands held healing power. They wanted their little ones to be caressed by those hands.

Touch. Our skin hungers for it. It appears that touch gets "under our skin" and makes its way to our hearts. It tells us that we are not alone. It assures us that we are loved. The Greek

61

word for touch can also be translated "to kindle" or "to light."
Touch. It kindles a fire in our flesh and puts a light in our eyes.
It warms us to the core. It keeps us alive. Perhaps Luke did
not need to describe Jesus blessing the babes. A tender touch
from a loving person was, in itself, a blessing.

As soon as we were born, we began to write the first chapter of the sexual story that we carry in our flesh to this day. It
started with touch. The self-touch that began *in utero* underwent further development at our birth. For the first time, we
felt the touch of someone else's hands on our flesh. That sensation of being held in the hands of another provided us with the
initial psychosexual encounter of our newborn life. With it we
began to learn, primarily through sensate experience, the first
lesson of sexuality: sexuality has to do with human contact.

Psychosexual development. From the beginning, it means
reverencing the sacred ground of our bodies. It means believing that flesh is a dwelling place of God and that all parts of
our bodies are worthy of blessing. It means trusting that the
words spoken by Jesus to the infants are also addressed to each
of us. It means letting the invitation given to the babes of the
first century be an invitation to our own embodied selves.

The Sexual Responses of the Newborn

It's a girl! Our arrival was announced with a proclamation of
our sexual identity. Before comments were made about our
dark curls or ruddy complexions, our sexual identities were
heralded. Before our parents counted our toes, they probably took careful note of our bodies to confirm us as sons or
daughters.

It's a boy! Our newborn bodies confirmed the announcement by making a sexual statement of their own. As males,
we might have been born with an erection. As females, we
displayed vaginal lubrication at birth. In addition, our genitals were engorged. Because these responses are attributed
to the high concentrations of pregnancy hormones present at
birth, there has been a tendency to dismiss them as temporary physiological events that have no real significance for us
as newborns.

In actuality, engorged genitals feel different from the way

they do when they are not engorged. Just as we had awareness of hunger, we also had sensate awareness of the feeling of energy that accompanied our biological sexual responses.

Our response to prenatal sex hormones is testimony that our sexuality was operative from the beginning, not as a set of physical organs that provided a convenient way to distinguish us as boys or girls, but as a powerful capacity for sexual responding.

Sexuality cannot be presumed to be inoperative in children and of consequence only for the adult who is ready to procreate. Rather, our sexuality is a dynamic source of energy from the first moments of our life, eager to allure us with its cosmic fire.

It's a girl! It's a boy! With the first recitation of these words, we began the transition from generic "babyness" to a real-life personal identity. No longer an "it," we were somebody, a boy or a girl. As the Vatican document so powerfully asserts, it is from sex that we receive the first aspect of a personal identity that will continue to evolve in its uniqueness as long as we live. And to the momentous announcement, our newborn bodies responded. We greeted the world with breath and a sexual response!

The Stages of Childhood
Psychosexual Development

What does the journey of psychosexual integration involve? What is its direction? Ultimately, if our development proceeds in a healthy fashion, we become adults who are capable of self-disclosive intimacy. Our sexual desires and behaviors will be integrated with well-tested communication skills, ethical values and sensitivities to other people. Immediately after our birth, however, self-disclosive intimacy was a faraway possibility, not an actuality. Instead of integration between the genital and interpersonal dimensions of our life, there was separation. Part of the lifelong task of our psychosexual development has been to bring the two together, to forge a connection between the raw, undisciplined bodily desires of infancy, and our fragile potential for forming relationships.

We can look at psychosexual development in greater detail by examining the cycles of awakening, exploring, and relating that we went through at different age periods:

- Sexual unawareness: birth to toddler
- Sexual awakening: toddler to early preschool
- Sexual socialization: early preschool to the onset of puberty

Phase I:

Sexual Unawareness: Birth to Toddler

During the first baby phase, which lasted until we were about eighteen months of age, the term "unawareness" refers to our cognitive inability to differentiate our physical experiences from one another. The good feelings we had in connection with being held and nursed, the release associated with elimination, the occasional sensation of pleasure in our genitals, or the relief brought about by a diaper change were all part of one great universal body comfort.

In our infancy, we were sexually "unaware" in another way. Any pleasurable genital sensations during this period were due to involuntary responses and not to any conscious attempt on our part to elicit them. In addition to the rhythmic physical responses discussed earlier, it was normal for us to have occasional pleasurable genital sensations when we were being nursed, cuddled, or bathed. Although we did not experience them as specifically "sexual," these autonomic responses to being tended and loved were ways that relationality and genitality were instinctively connected. The baby who continues to associate comforting body responses with human loving will one day be the adult who does the same.

The sexual unawareness characteristic of our newborn lives gradually gave way to an increasing sense of consciousness of ourselves. One dimension of this advancing level of psychosexual development began taking place as we came to know and attain mastery over our own flesh, and the other happened as we learned to trust and bond with our caretakers.

Early Psychosexual Development and Body Touch

The sensate experiences of our flesh were a critical vehicle for learning about sexuality at this stage of development. As newborns, we were instinctively eager to continue to know our flesh. Our mouths, our eyes, our ears, our noses, our skin brought the tastes, sights, sounds, smells and the feel of our world close. The gradual accumulation of knowledge via sensate experience enabled us to attain a sense of control over our bodies and an increasing awareness of the physical world. It is from our body that we formed our first messages about sexuality. The early experiences of our flesh gave us the raw material for the first chapter of our postnatal sexual story. If we were handled gently, if our bodily needs were well attended, if our attempts at body exploration and genital touching were respected, we probably learned that our bodies were a good and safe place in which to live.

Early Psychosexual Development and the Touch of the Heart

Let the children come to me! Learning to come to others, to approach, to trust, to be touched was a central part of our early psychosexual development. The arduous process of learning how to initiate and maintain social, emotional bonds with others started when we first made eye contact with our mothers. It continued as we studied the facial cues of our caretakers and began to mimic them. Eventually, we learned to match facial expressions to certain key emotions. We learned to attract attention, and to desire the presence of those who were familiar and comforting to us. Already then we were moving toward achieving the ultimate purpose of human sexuality as a " . . . union of life and of love . . . " (Pastoral Constitution on the Church in the Modern World).

While the little game of "peek-a-boo" was yet a long way from self-disclosive intimacy, it was a first step toward it. It was one of the ways we gained familiarity in saying, "I see you" and "You can see me." This process of seeing and being seen, at ever increasing levels, was part of our early journey toward intimacy. Our attachments to a special blanket, a stuffed animal, a favorite toy, were also ways that we experimented with attachment. Through them we learned to hold things to our hearts, to have preferences, and to feel fondness. We also learned to count on the presence and permanence of the things we found dear. This learning was preparing us for the day when we would exchange a teddy bear for our first real friend.

The Occurrence of Genital Fondling During Infancy

Our first smile. Our first word. Our first step. Ever so gradually we entered more fully into the world of relationships. Each of these achievements marked a certain milestone for us and was probably greeted with fanfare and encouragement. Yet there was another area of relational skill we were attaining that probably passed without notice. Related to body mastery, it involved the gradual *coming to consciousness* of the energy of our sexuality. Little by little, the pleasant autonomic genital sensations of our infancy became more differentiated from our other bodily sensations. By about six months of age, we might have discovered that we could produce a nice feeling of pleasure by fondling our genitals.

Between twelve and eighteen months, we became capable of experiencing a rudimentary form of orgasm. Although some of us engaged in occasional genital fondling, culminating in orgasm, not all of us did. The varieties of sexual intensity and interest characteristic of normal adults seem to be manifested already in babies.

Studies show that the physiological pattern of arousal for the toddler roughly parallels that of adults. It is accompanied by rhythmic body movement, an increasing respiratory rate, a faster heartbeat, and elevated blood pressure, followed by release. However, the *psychological* components are quite different. Babies do not have the same kinds of emotional feelings with orgasm that are had by the normal adolescent or adult. During childhood, orgasm is not connected to feelings of arousal for a particular person, but rather to a kind of cosmic experience of solitary pleasure. The focus of self-pleasuring for the infant is genitality as opposed to relationality. While the infant does have a primitive association between genital pleasure and human attachment, this association is still outside conscious awareness.

While baby books usually have a place to note "Baby's First Word" or the date for "Baby's First Step," none of them have a page to record the sounds and footsteps of baby's sexual awakening. Yet this often unobtrusive "waking up" is no less important to our developing capacity for adult love than were the communication and mobility achievements that were being welcomed with such enthusiasm around the same time. Uttering "dada" and "mama" have helped us find the words for mature love. Toddling alone from the couch to the chair has become the independent steps of our adult decision making. And no less significant, the tentative experience of self-initiated genital pleasuring gave us the framework for increasingly disciplined sexual behavior and choices.

The Significance of Genital Fondling During Infancy and Childhood

The genital touching that most of us engaged in sometime during infancy served an important role in our growth. First, it enabled us to know our flesh and to solidify awareness of our body boundaries. Second, it acquainted us with the erotic potential of our bodies in a gradual and safe way. And finally, it provided us with a sense of "ownership" of our sexual energies.

Self-touch was the primary way that we became familiar with our body. It introduced us to the feel, position, and uniqueness of our genitals. This contributed to our sense of body comfort. For those of us who might have been allowed to suck our fingers and play with our toes but were discouraged from touching our genitals, we might have learned to feel some alienation from this part of our body.

The most secure way for us to become aware of and comfortable with the sexual energies of our bodies is, quite literally, "at our own hands." When we initiated genital touch ourselves and progressed tentatively and gradually to more active genital stimulation, we began to experience ourselves as the agent of our own decision making. We were the ones in charge. We were able to produce sensations that had a clear beginning and ending. We could engage in actions with our own bodies that had a predictable outcome. With every self-initiated pleasurable experience, we came to know that our sexual energy was not a force outside our control, or an alien power that did not belong. Rather, it was a containable energy, an obedient power, willing to be tamed. Long before such an energy could be shared in mature lovemaking with another, it had to be befriended in our own bodies. Before a gift can be shared, it must be known.

If our early efforts to explore our bodies were responded to warmly, our initial encounters with embodiment were positive. Our precognitive experience taught us that flesh is friendly, that we can trust it. If that was our experience, we accomplished another segment of the journey toward becoming incarnate. We were ready for the next step.

Phase II:

Sexual Awakening: Toddler to Early Preschool

While the sexual awakening characteristic of the second phase of childhood psychosexual development is one among many sexual awakenings in the healthy human person, it has the special distinction of being the earliest. It signals that sexuality has now come to consciousness.

Somewhere between the ages of eighteen and twenty-four months, we became aware that our genitals had a uniqueness about them that compelled special attention. It was as though a new "ah ah" moment had occurred. The heightened interest focused on genitality during our toddler phase was occasioned by several critical developmental tasks in which we were absorbed: *acquisition of language, toilet training*, and *formation of gender identity*.

Acquisition of Language

When we became toddlers, we experienced an explosion of information that can be likened to that which Helen Keller had when she first learned the sign for water. The fresh cool liquid running through her fingers finally had a name! Now she could associate a wide variety of things with labels that were distinct. No longer a prisoner of silence, she had a way to communicate, to connect with her world.

For ourselves as toddlers, the discovery of words meant much the same thing. The acquisition of a language, the magic of names, whether by words or signs, triggered our movement from ignorance to understanding, from separation to connection, from confusion to meaning. It gave us a new tool for future self-disclosure.

Soon after we began to say our first words, our parents began the naming game. This involved teaching us a name for the parts of our bodies, or at least the parts they were comfortable saying! A friend shared this story, illustrating a common omission:

> When our daughter, Maria, was just beginning to talk, my wife's mother visited us from the east coast. One day, as she was dressing Maria, we heard her give the following vocabulary lesson as she pointed to our little girl's various body parts:
>
> "This is your eye. This is your nose. This is your ear. This is your mouth. This is your arm. This is your tummy. This is your knee...." With that, Maria, who had previously played the naming game with us, pulled her grandmother's hand up from her knee, touched it lightly to her genitals and said: "Dis gina!" With that, grandma's face reddened and her body visibly tightened. She quickly changed the subject, dressed Maria, and took her to the park.

While Grandma certainly did not intend it, she indirectly conveyed an unhelpful message to young Maria about sexuality. The message might have been "we don't talk about sex" or "your genitals do not have a name." In either case, Maria's earlier healthier parenting allowed her to name her "gina" and thus claim it as belonging to her body. This is just one step on the way toward Maria's growing ability to take responsibility for her sexuality and for helping her establish an increasing level of body comfort. Although Maria would not be able to articulate it, being able to give a name to her genitals (at least at the two-year-old level), is already helping her establish a boundary around her sexuality and to reverence her genitals with a name.

Toilet Training

When we were toddlers, as we gained control over elimination we experienced a growing sense of accomplishment and pride in the part of our bodies where these functions occurred.

Few people today would trace the majority of the psychological problems that can afflict the human person back to faulty toilet training, as Freud is sometimes credited with doing. Still, the fact remains that toilet training is a sensitive time in a young child's life. When successes are affirmed and "accidents" are met with understanding and encouragement, the child's self-esteem, feeling of competence, and ability to handle failure without loss of face are enhanced. Because of the toddler's tendency to fuse elimination experiences with genital ones, the positive feelings associated with toilet training will be transferred, largely on an unconscious level, to the child's developing sexual identity. Whatever positive or negative associations occur here will in some way influence adult sexuality.

Gender Identity

In addition to language acquisition and toilet training, our growing consciousness of our genitals had another, perhaps more compelling, reason. Put simply, noticing them was central to learning whether we were boys or girls. When we were two, our male and female bodies were essentially identical except for our differing sexual organs. Achieving a stable sense of gender identity presupposed that we knew which set of sexual parts we had. While we have stressed that sexuality cannot be confined to gender labels, it is the place we had to begin.

It was not only our own genitals that drew our interest as young children. If we had occasion to view our peers, siblings, or parents unclothed, we were fascinated by their bodies as well. Staring, pointing, touching, and attempting to pronounce the names of sexual parts, whether our own or someone else's, were all part of the normal way in which we came to a sense of the permanence of our own maleness or femaleness.

Psychosexual Development and the Growth of Body Comfort

Toddlers are proud of their bodies and delightfully at home with them. Not yet self-conscious about nakedness, they experience their bodies as their most prized possession. This is the age of "youthful streakers" who run naked into the living room in the midst of company. Children usually receive a different reaction coming forth unclothed than they do fully attired. They quickly begin to learn that there is something about uncovered genitals that is not true of bare feet in quite the same way. This adds to their own observation that their genitals are quite interesting and serves to increase their awareness that there is an importance attributed to them that makes them particularly worthy of covering and protecting.

The comfort that young children have with physical nakedness has a significance that reaches beyond the fact that they are not yet self-conscious. Each of us is born with a desire to reveal ourselves to another. We learn to do this in gradually progressive ways. Long before we are able to share the depth of our "inmost selves" with a beloved one, we reveal ever-increasing dimensions of who we are to others. As two-year-olds, we are ready to go beyond "peek-a-boo" and spontaneously show our bodies — to let others see more of us. Later, we will experiment with other forms of self-revelation: We will state our thoughts, make known our feelings, share the vulnerability of our hearts. But for now, at age two, our self-disclosure is limited to what we know best: the miracle of our flesh.

Little Darin's story provides an example of how all the tasks of this phase of childhood psychosexual development interweave with each other and, we hope, culminate in greater integration.

When Darin was two-and-a-half years old, his Aunt Jean visited the family from out of town. Darin was so excited over her visit that he had "an accident." While Jean and her sister visited, Darin's father took his young son to the nursery to change his wet training pants. Within minutes, Darin ran squealing into the living room wearing only his socks. He planted himself in front of his aunt and said proudly: "Auntie Jean, you want to see my penis?" Though somewhat stunned and amused, his aunt's response matched Darin's enthusiasm about this newly named part of his anatomy. "Why, Darin," she smiled, "that's a very nice penis!" Darin looked pleased and ran out of the room. Two minutes later, he was back, still wearing only his socks. This time, his attention was on another new and exciting part of the world he was learning to label. "Auntie Jean," he exclaimed, "you want to see my truck?" His aunt responded as warmly as before. "Oh, Darin, what a nice truck!" After several more trips in and out of the nursery to show and name his most prized possessions, the game ended. Darin was dressed and retreated quietly to a corner of the living room to page through a book. He had been affirmed. He had gotten the attention he needed for his newfound ability to know the names of things.

Had the adults overreacted, either by laughing and trying to prolong his antics or, conversely, by scolding him, the outcome could have been entirely different. Very likely, his attention would not have shifted to his truck, but remained fixed where it was. When children's normal interest in sex is exploited, punished, ridiculed, or diminished, their attention tends to stay focused there. Worse, if the punishment is severe or occurs repeatedly, they may learn to associate sex with shame or anxiety, thus developing harmful attitudes toward sexuality.

Psychosexual development does not proceed automatically; it requires the solid ground of self-awareness and self-acceptance. The more toddlers have experienced genitality as a positive, comfortable, and affirmed part of their identity, the better equipped they will be to carry it responsibly into the future. Children for whom sexual awakening has been a frightening, traumatic, or punitive experience already experience their sexuality as wounded. These wounds will usually express themselves one way or another later in life.

Phase III:

Psychosexual Socialization: Preschool to Puberty

Let the children come to me. Do not hinder them. To such belongs the kingdom of God. The evangelists used a story about children to illustrate the kind of innocence required to enter the reign of God. God's kingdom is not about status, importance, or knowledge. Perfection is not an entrance requirement. What is? Look at a child. See the incompleteness. Feel the vulnerability. Watch the eagerness to learn. The reign of God is about spilt milk and skinned knees. It has to do with happy giggles and toothless grins, with falling down and getting up again.

Childhood is an image for the reign of God. Childhood has to do with growing, changing, exploring, discovering. Childhood is a time when socks don't have to match and coloring outside the lines is allowed. There is something inherent in childhood that gives permission for mistakes and makes room for development. Probably nowhere is this more important than in the third phase of childhood psychosexual development — the time when social skills are being refined, young bodies are becoming more coordinated, and ethical standards for relationships are being introduced. Childhood is a signpost for the reign of God.

To Such Belongs the Kingdom of God

Somewhere around the age of three or four, we entered a period of psychosexual development characterized by a quiet deepening. This occurred both in regard to our bodies as well as to our relational capacities. It was a time for the sexual and social realities of our lives to become more comfortably connected.

By this time, we had learned that our genitals were the "private parts" of our bodies and were normally kept covered. We had probably also learned that touching or rubbing our genitals, using sexual words, or being obvious about sexual interest was not something people do in public. Although we remained quite interested in sexual matters, we were now becoming more careful about showing it. We learned to contain our curiosity, to be more surreptitious about our interests.

The advent of embarrassment around anything pertaining to nakedness or sexual talk marks the beginning of this phase for many children. This may be manifested by giggling, feigning disinterest, or showing visible signs of discomfort when anything sexual is discussed. For many children, though not all of them, entrance into the stage of psychosexual socialization is also characterized by an increased sense of modesty when bathing, dressing, or using the bathroom. Nakedness becomes attached to privacy. This new self-consciousness around sexuality is a result of our awareness that we are sexual and that being sexual is invested with mystery — mystery that is deserving of care.

Sexuality, Hormones, and the Childhood Search for Connection

"He's only seven, but he seems to touch himself more than his nine-year-old brother. Maybe his hormones are just more active." These words spoken by a young mother to her child's pediatrician betray a common misunderstanding. The popular assumption that sex hormones have a proportionate relationship to sex drive is faulty. Although some relationship does exist in adults (although not a proportionate one), the same is not true of children.

The bodies of children are relatively dormant in terms of the sex hormones. After a surge of testosterone about the second week of life, little boys do not produce any more of this male sex hormone until the advent of puberty. Little girls do not begin estrogen production until the same time. Still, young children maintain a capacity for genital arousal and have varying degrees of interest in self-stimulation throughout childhood.

This biological reality suggests that the sexual responses of children are more personal and social in nature than they are hormonal. Children are not driven by high levels of sex hormones to fondle themselves. The occasional self-pleasuring and bodily exploration associated with prepubescent children are part of their natural need to know themselves and their bodies. They look because they are curious. They touch because they seek familiarity through contact. They rub because they are instinctively drawn to the sensate pleasure that their little bodies house. They explore their flesh because some place deep inside them seeks further incarnation.

Sociosexual Play: Rehearsal for Adult Love

"You be the daddy. I'll be the mommy." An important aspect of psychosexual development begins during this period. It is directed toward preparation for adult interpersonal sharing. It is called "sociosexual play," and it coincides with the socialized play that commences around the age of three or four.

Play is the practice field for real life. It provides safe, well-paced opportunities for us to rehearse the skills needed for adult relationships. Through play we "try on" the feelings and behaviors of those whose roles we are playing. This is one of the ways we learn empathy — an important quality for adult friendship. Play also provides us with opportunities for taking turns, negotiating roles, and setting boundaries in relationships. It is also the place where self-disclosure becomes more purposeful and sophisticated. The urge to know and be known eventually moves beyond "peek-a-boo."

Prior to socialized play, as toddlers we played side by side, each absorbed in our own separate pursuits. Our sex play during this time involved the solitary self-pleasuring discussed earlier. However, once we began to interact, to share toys, to talk to each other, and to become involved in the same activity, our sex play underwent a change that corresponded to our level of advancing social skill. Curiosity about the genitals of the other, expressed when we were younger by pointing or staring, develops into occasional, mutual exploration. Even though we might not have clear memories of it, the "you show me yours and I'll show you mine" games of childhood probably occurred to some degree in each of our lives.

The critical word during this important stage is "mutual." The tentative glance into another's underpants, the quick touch, the apprehension around "getting caught" all became *shared*. What had been a very solitary interest now took the first step toward what would eventually become the capacity for the full psychosexual mutuality of the mature adult. If these first joint experiences with sexual mutuality through play were enjoyable and successful, we would have accomplished another goal toward our ongoing psychosexual integration. We would eventually come to know, through the experience of play, that *sex involves sharing*, that we are competent to handle it, and that the excitement surrounding it is *relational* as well as physical.

The hesitant, often furtive sex play of a couple of four-year-olds needs to become more secure and focused as the child matures. Playing "doctor," playing "house," paging through *National Geographic* with its acceptable pictures of naked South Sea islanders, and secretly giggling over "naughty" words and jokes are common ways that we might have experienced more prolonged and organized forms of sociosexual play as we grew older.

Often, the healthy sex play of children is not directly pursued, but is the outcome of other forms of play that involve clothing changes or body contact. Locker rooms, camping trips, or slumber parties sometimes provide an occasion for children to continue to use play as the setting to explore the mutual revelation of their bodies. The following story, shared by a co-worker, is a good example:

> Several of my cousins were visiting, and we were in the guest bedroom, preparing to change to go swimming. Initially, there was an argument about who would get to use the room to change first, the boys or the girls. This turned into a contest, with someone suggesting that whoever took their clothes off first could claim the room for the other members of their gender. There was a lot of giggling and daring one another to be the first to undress. Gradually, we each began to remove various articles of clothing, and eventually there were a half dozen eight-, nine-, and ten- year-olds darting naked about the room throwing their underpants at each other. The commotion attracted the attention of my mother, who opened the door, sent the boys to an upstairs bedroom, and told us all to put our swimming suits on and get to the pool.

The act of showing one's body to the beloved in a relaxed and unself-conscious way doesn't just happen as the automatic by-product of a marriage ceremony or a love commitment. It is prepared for slowly, over time, in the many different childhood games described above. When children engage in the awkward display of their naked bodies to their peers in sometimes silly, usually self-conscious play, they gain a measure of experience in self-revelation. The mutuality, the satisfaction of curiosity, the freedom of choice to participate or not, the shared excitement, the fun, the safe context, the sense of personal control in pacing the activity, all contribute to a child's growing sense of sexual competence and experience. One day the awkwardness about being naked before another will be diminished, and the game will give way to the adult capacity for comfortable physical sharing.

The Essential Conditions of Healthy Sociosexual Play

When we present workshops on the topic of psychosexual development, we frequently meet persons who have questions about the normalcy of particular situations they have encountered in the sexual behaviors of children. Often they are concerned parents and teachers who want to be sure that the activities of the children in their care are not harmful to them. Sometimes they are people remembering their own childhood sexual experiences and wondering if what they did was "normal."

The sexual play of childhood is considered healthy and normal only when it occurs *willingly* among children who are *peers* and when the type of activity is *age appropriate*. While the definition of peer can occasionally be nuanced, they are usually regarded as those who are within about two years of each other's ages and are in the same stage of psychosexual development. "Age appropriate" refers to the type of activity involved. Normally, the sexual behavior of children centers around looking, touching, and talking.

Whenever young children engage in sexual behaviors that they would not ordinarily discover by themselves or know about from within a child's frame of reference, there is reason for concern. Likewise, if sexual activity among peers is coerced, evokes fear, or involves acting out previous experiences of sexual abuse, the activity does not qualify as play. Whenever any of the following conditions are present in sexual behavior among children, the behavior needs to be stopped, quickly and with care, and the child's pediatrician or school counselor ought to be consulted:

- participants who are not peers
- absence of mutuality
- penetration of bodily orifices
- preoccupation or obsession with sex play
- sexual precociousness (sexual knowledge beyond their years)
- presence of violence or infliction of pain
- use of manipulation or pressure to participate
- initiation of the play by an adolescent or adult
- sex play that is very obvious, or done in public places
- presence of fear or shame around normal childhood sex play

In determining the appropriateness of sexual behavior among children, it is important to consider that many children today have access to sexual information in the media that was not available to us when we were growing up. It is not uncommon for today's children to see erotic sexual imagery that is beyond their capacity to understand emotionally. We can prevent our children from viewing material that is inappropriate for them when they are at home, but we cannot always control what a playmate might introduce them to or what they might see at a friend's house. Maintaining open communication with our children, being aware of their activities, and knowing as much as possible about the home life of their playmates can help assure an environment that promotes healthy psychosexual growth, instead of hindering it.

Do Not Hinder Them

Jesus wasn't talking about psychosexual development when he spoke these words. He was making sure that the children coming to him to be touched would not be prevented from doing so. He was trying to remove any obstacles that would hinder the babes from having access to him and to the holy caress that would bless their bodies and nourish their hearts.

Do not hinder them. Do not prevent them from experiencing healthy human contact. Do not stop them from seeking affirmation for their flesh. Do not subject them to rejection. Do not stand in the way of their journey. We can hear these words echoed against the backdrop of all our efforts to grow as human persons. We can let the words of Jesus to his disciples be a challenge for our own relationships with children. Do not hinder them. They belong.

Our work with our clients continues to teach us that one of the primary places that we can be hindered is in the area of sexuality. Touch can curse as well as bless. Play can turn into abuse. Our efforts to become incarnate can be hindered.

Let the Children Grow

Erchomai. Most of the time when it is used in the Christian scriptures, this Greek word is translated "come." It means movement forward. It suggests a journey, a transition from one place to another. Almost always it implies a decision, a choice to set out in search of something. It is not surprising that the word can also be translated "grow." Let the children come to me. Let them move forward. Let them *grow.* Let them set out on a journey that will bring them into contact with someone who knows something about incarnation.

Psychosexual development is about incarnation. It's about entering flesh. It's about touching and being touched. It's about learning to love and be loved. It's about playing. It's about making sure that we never grow too old to run into someone's arms and receive a blessing.

QUESTIONS FOR REFLECTION AND SHARING

These questions have been designed to help you personalize what you have just read. They are a way of getting in touch with your own story, of exploring what in you needs further growth or healing. Do not feel that you have to respond to all of them. Also, you may wish to reflect on them over several occasions. You may find it helpful to spend some time in prayer with them, to record your responses in your journal, or in some cases to share your responses with a close friend or significant other.

1. What "body memories," stories, or imaginings do you have about how you were held as a baby? Nursed? Tended? What relationship do you recognize between these early experiences and your current level of comfort with body touch? Giving and receiving affection? Feeling physically needy or physically comfortable?

2. What baby pictures have you seen of yourself? What do you think/feel your experience was like as a baby? Or what was it like to be a baby in your family when you were born?

3. What do you recall about your play experiences? Playmates? Favorite toys? Games? How do these relate to your interests in people today? Enjoyments?

4. What memories do you have around self-pleasuring (masturbation)? Childhood sex play? Body exploration?

5. Were there any traumas during your childhood? Sexual abuse? Being "caught" during sex play or body exploration? Any punishments related to sexual behavior?

6. What do you remember, or what have you been told, about coming to understand your gender identity (maleness or femaleness)? How were boys and girls valued in your family? Treated differently? What were the family rules for "boy behavior" and "girl behavior"?

7. What messages did you receive about sex and sexuality as a child from parents? Siblings? Friends? Church? School? What effect did these messages have then? Now? Which ones were helpful? Not helpful?

8. How do you think your childhood experiences of sexuality express themselves today in your:

- level of body comfort and self-esteem?

- feelings of sexual arousal?

- interior "self-talk" about your sexuality?

- ways of attempting to connect with others as a man or a woman?

- degree and type of sexual guilt? Discomfort? Comfort?

6

GROWING IN WISDOM AND GRACE

Psychosexual Development in Adolescence

And Jesus grew in wisdom, in stature, and in grace with God and men.

— Luke 2:52

Luke is the only evangelist who gives us a portrait of Jesus as an adolescent. From a human perspective, it is a brief but revealing glimpse of a young Jewish boy emerging from childhood into his first awareness of adult identity.

According to tradition, when a Jewish male reached the age of twelve, he was expected to begin observing the Torah as an adult. This included making the pilgrimages to Jerusalem for the important religious feasts. In Luke's narrative, Jesus is drawn to the teachers of the Law, who sat in the shade of the temple galleries, teaching and dialoguing with groups of pilgrims. When the feast ends, Jesus remains in Jerusalem, while his family and friends begin their trip back to Nazareth. After a day's journey, his parents discover his absence and anxiously come in search of him. When they find him, there is a mixture of relief, confusion, and concern.

There are also questions. Questions that have probably resonated, in one way or another, with parents and adolescents of every succeeding generation, including the present. Why have you done this to us? Why were you looking for me? Didn't you realize? Didn't you know?

Over the centuries in Christian devotional life, this story came to be known by an interesting title. It was called the "Losing of the Christ Child in the Temple." This title is a telling commentary on our human uneasiness with "growing up." It is clear from Luke's account that Jesus was *not* lost. On the contrary, without asking permission and without telling his parents, he freely chose to stay in Jerusalem. If anything, it would be more correct to say that Jesus was *finding himself* in the temple. He was following his vocational call, asserting his freedom and independence. He was beginning to claim his life as a man.

This last statement is worth emphasizing. Jesus was *beginning* to claim his life as an adult. Growing up is not an event, but a process. We begin to "leave home" long before we physically move out of the house. Thus Luke tells us that Jesus returned to Nazareth to live "under the authority" of his parents, and the story concludes with this observation: "And Jesus grew in wisdom, in stature, and in grace with God and men" (2:52).

The central challenge of our teenage years is contained in these simple words. It is a time for us to grow in wisdom, stature, and grace with God and others. We cannot assume, of course, that Luke was intending to give us a "spirituality of adolescence" in this pericope. That would be a misuse of the gospel text. All the same, this story does give us a striking snapshot of Jesus at a crucial turning point in his life. It is a story of passage and transition, of setting out on the human quest. In one way or another, these experiences resonate in each of our lives. They are the "stuff" of the human journey. They reflect the dreams and demands of moving from childhood to adult responsibility. Looked at from this perspective, this story can serve as a starting point for our reflections on the central tasks of adolescent growth and psychosexual development.

Adolescence and the Human Condition

Recently, a participant in a workshop told us that she felt "ill-at-ease" when we spoke of Jesus as an adolescent. She is probably not alone. Many of us are uncomfortable thinking of Jesus as a teenager. We prefer to see him either as the infant at Bethlehem or the mature rabbi who travelled the roads of Palestine.

Why is this? Perhaps because we can't imagine why God would get so "involved" in the human condition with its physical and emotional transitions. Perhaps we are uncomfortable with our own humanity.

More specifically, perhaps our uneasiness has something to do with our sexuality. It is relatively easy for us to recite the creed, affirming our belief that Jesus was both the Son of God and the son of Mary, that he is divine and at the same time fully human. This is the language of doctrine. It is correct, but somewhat distant from our personal experience. But when we explore the implications of these creedal statements, we are likely to feel less comfortable.

What does it mean to say that Jesus was fully human? Did he experience puberty like the rest of us? Did his parents notice when he began to grow facial hair? Did he feel sexual desire? The level of our uneasiness in asking these questions may be a good indicator of how at home we are with our humanity. And his.

We begin this exploration of the adolescent years with a desire to affirm this challenging and hope-filled time in our lives. This is the season when our dreams are born and our visions are claimed. These are the years of risk and self-discovery. These are the times of coming to know the intensity of our feelings and the soaring desires of our hearts. With all its uncertainty, anxiety, confusion, and awkwardness, adolescence is nevertheless a sacred adventure into life.

In most ancient cultures, young people were initiated into adulthood through sacred rituals, referred to as "rites of passage." This initiation was followed by a period of apprenticeship during which their elders taught them the necessary skills for their roles.

In many contemporary cultures, this fundamental reverence for youth has been replaced with a strange mixture of fascination and fear. In its etymological roots, the term "adolescent" carries the positive meaning of "growing up" or "maturing." In our time it has come to mean almost the opposite — a lack of maturity, an inability to be responsible, an awkward, inconsistent state of mind.

Part of the reason for this negative understanding of adolescence may be due to our own painful memories. As adults we often tend to focus on the negative images of our growing up. Perhaps we need to begin by being more gentle with our own memories of growing up and with our stumbling attempts to understand and cope with our changing sexual feelings.

The Second Awakening

In the journey toward maturity, most living organisms move through a period of dramatic transformation — a time that some scientists refer to as the "critical phase" of growth. During these turning points, the life-force appears to leap forward to a new level of actualization. In our human journey, adolescence is clearly the "critical phase" in our growth. Next to our physical birth and death, it is probably the most dramatic time of change in our lives.

Earlier, we proposed two ways of looking at our psychosexual development. The first, illustrated in Figure 1, describes our growth in terms of stages that are chronological and linear; the second, illustrated in Figure 2, emphasizes the recurring and unfinished cycles of our growth. It might be helpful at this point to recall that this second model also describes a certain "rhythm" in these recurring cycles. This rhythm usually follows a motif of *awakening* and *exploring*, followed by a deeper level of interpersonal *relating*.

The first dramatic expression of this rhythm took place in our infancy. During our adolescent years this cycle of growth recurs, this time with even more intensity, since it is now more conscious and self-directed. Every aspect of our personality — physical, emotional, cognitional, psychological, spiritual — is experiencing a new level of being alive. We might call it our "second awakening." This is in turn followed by the desire to know and explore this newly emerging vitality and eventually to channel it into mature forms of friendship and love.

Leaving Home: The Background Music

Developmental psychologists usually describe two distinct movements in our journey through adolescence. The first and earlier stage begins with the onset of puberty and lasts until we are approximately fifteen or sixteen years of age. This phase is characterized by a new and intense time of pushing toward independence from our parents and caretakers. It hearkens back to the first stirrings of assertiveness that occurred when we were young children saying our defiant "no" to the wishes or suggestions of our parents.

Sometimes this push toward independence takes the form of tension, confrontation, or even open rebellion toward our parents and teachers. At other times, it is a silent claiming of our inner truth without necessarily engaging in confrontation. It is a mistaken notion to think that most of us achieve our initial grasp of adult identity through open rebellion. Many of us simply make this transition quietly and deeply, without fanfare and without fuss.

At the same time that we are striving to claim our own psychic "turf," we still experience a tug toward emotional dependence. The result is a fascinating ritual, a kind of psychic dance between our desire for separate identity and our lingering need for assurance. At one moment we are arguing for our right to have a separate bank account and the privilege of choosing our own forms of entertainment. In the next moment, we are asking our parents for money to put in the account and transportation to go spend it.

During the second phase of psychosocial development this tension between independence and dependence will slowly be resolved — at least under healthy conditions — in the direction of adult identity. Our maturing self manifests itself through vocational choices as well as decisions about how we will or will not express our sexual and relational interests.

This overarching task of leaving home is the "background music" for the drama of adolescence. It is the framework in which our psychosexual journey unfolds during this phase of our lives. It should come as no surprise that this is often a time of uncertainty and anxiety. Like Jesus in the Lucan story, we are beginning to claim our future. We are following the ancient call to leave a familiar place — even if it may not be a particularly safe or healthy place — to set out toward the unknown and the unfamiliar. Setting out into the unknown can be frightening at any time in our lives. During adolescence

this anxiety is heightened since it is not only our external sur-
roundings that are undergoing transformation, but also the
inner geography of our physical and emotional responses.

Phase I:

Sexual Fantasizing

The power of imagination is an essential dimension of human
life in all its stages of growth. We cannot live on data alone.
The real stuff of life is made up of dreams and visions. In order
to grow, our psyches need to have room to play and to expand
their horizons. We need space to nurture dreams and to "waste
time" with stories, games, and roles that engage our imagina-
tions and motivate our quest for adventure. Imagination is
the inner wellspring of creativity and relational energy. Our
day dreams as children become the friendships, the covenantal
bonds, the inventions, the novels, and the projects of our adult
years. As these images and intuitions become more mature,
they flower into real relationships. Sometimes they become the
developed capacity to write poetry, paint masterpieces, com-
pose symphonies, and create scientific revolutions. Equally
as important, they may be expressed in caring for the sick,
teaching children, or building houses.

Rehearsal for Relationships

What does the power of the imagination have to do with
adolescent sexual fantasies? Why is sexual fantasizing such an
important part of our ability to mature in our relational lives?

In addition to the multiplicity of physical, hormonal
changes that are taking place during our teenage years, there is
also a significant transformation taking place on the emotional
and psychic level. One of these is a shift in the direction and focus of our sexual energy. In the infant and child, for the most
part, sexual responsiveness is undifferentiated and free flow-
ing. It is like the energy of cosmic allurement that we spoke of
in chapter 1. During adolescence this undifferentiated energy
begins to become more focused and relational. It begins to become attached to persons, whether real or imaginary. The most

important human faculty that assists this "personalization" of sexual energy is our ability to *fantasize*. Sexual fantasy is the human capacity to explore our relational horizons. It is an interior and imaginative way of engaging the human need to reach out to other people. It is *rehearsal for relationships*.

This is not to suggest that the role of fantasy is limited only to the adolescent stage of our growth. When we were children, we occupied ourselves with daydreams and engaged in many other elaborate forms of imaginative play. Fantasy continues to play an important role throughout our adult lives as well. What makes the adolescent form of fantasy so important is that for the first time it is more explicitly focused on our sexual attraction to other people. Sexual fantasy is our deep, intuitive way of preparing for mature love by picturing it in our minds and hearts.

Male-Female Differences in Sexual Fantasizing

Research seems to indicate that there are characteristic differences between the sexual fantasies of women and men. For the most part males tend to focus on physical appearance and bodily attractiveness. The content of their fantasies typically involves experiences that precede or lead to genital forms of intimacy. As a group men also tend to find visual stimuli to be a significant source of sexual interest and arousal.

On the other hand, women's sexual fantasies tend to be more romantic and relational. They may involve images that include physical intimacy, but their focus is more often centered around romantic settings such as dancing, walking in the sunset, having an intimate conversation, or being held in a caring way.

The Ethical Issue

We cannot explore the healthy role of sexual fantasy without addressing what has been called "impure thoughts" or "lusting in the heart." Many of us were taught that anyone who deliberately welcomes or "entertains" images, feelings, or thoughts about sexual matters is committing a grave sin. The sixth and ninth commandments were usually cited as a basis for this ethical teaching, as well as the words of Jesus: "If a man looks at a woman with lust, he has already committed adultery with her in his heart" (Mt 5:28).

Is there a way that we can resolve the apparent tension between healthy psychosexual development, on the one hand, and the demands of ethical teaching on the other? How can sexual fantasy be important for our relational growth and at the same time a potential threat to our moral integrity?

There are several historical and theological factors that converge around this issue of sexual thoughts, feelings, and images. Some of these factors are positive; they affirm our sexuality, even as they call us to "purity of heart." They reflect the core of our ethical tradition and enable us to clarify the difference between healthy sexual fantasies and inappropriate or morally objectionable ways of thinking. On the other hand, there are other historical factors in this discussion that are less positive and helpful. Let's examine both aspects.

On the positive side, we have inherited an emphasis in the Hebrew and Christian scriptures on human interiority as the basis for authentic ethical action. The "heart" — the deepest inner attitude of the human person — is the font from which all our external actions flow. Christian ethics places its priority on the quality of inner thoughts and feelings in contrast to mere external observance of the law (see Mt 15:1–20).

A second affirming influence from our religious heritage is the emphasis on the inherent goodness of the human person. From the earlier biblical vision to the contemporary church's social teaching, we encounter a common thread of reverence for what Pope John Paul II refers to as "the radical dignity of the human person." Finally, we have also inherited a strong incarnational basis for our ethical tradition, the respect we are called to have for the sacredness of our flesh. Both Judaism and Christianity are "creation centered" religions; they are committed to the fundamental goodness of the universe as it has unfolded from the creative hand of God and as it is imaged in the creation of woman and man. Flesh may be fragile and mortal, and at times wounded and broken, but it is also precious and filled with the mystery and goodness of the divine.

On the negative side, we recognize that Christianity has been persistently influenced by various forms of Gnosticism —

a belief system that looks with suspicion on our bodily needs and with outright disdain toward our sexual interests. This ideology has been expressed in many ways through the centuries with inevitably the same result: a fear of the body and sexuality, a suspicion of women, and a flight from authentic human intimacy.

Instead of viewing sexual fantasy as a healthy part of our human journey toward maturity, this attitude displays a neurotic fear of sexual thoughts, images, and desires. More often than not, the result of such thinking is an "obsessive compulsive" response to sexuality. Frequently, it manifests itself in one of two destructive extremes: either a repressed, rigid stance toward human feelings and relationships; or an addictive, even deviant fixation with sexual experience. In either case, this attitude of suspicion and fear is hardly conducive to psychosexual integration.

What conclusions can we draw from this brief summary of historical and theological factors? If sexual fantasy is a normal part of our psychosexual growth, how are we to interpret the meaning of "lust" and "impure" thoughts?

The answer to these questions lies in our ability to find a creative balance between nature and grace, between human wholeness and the call to holiness, between psychological health and the moral demands of the gospel.

Sexual feelings, desires, and images originate as spontaneous expressions of our growth toward relational maturity. Like other human needs, such as hunger, thirst, and security, they are in themselves good, or at least ethically neutral. It is our inner attitude toward them — the manner in which we consciously approach them — that gives them moral "weight" or value. The sin of gluttony does not mean that food or hunger is evil, nor does greed imply that having material possessions is wrong.

In the same way, lust is a serious sin, not because there is something evil about sexuality, but because, like all other human emotions, we can assume a manipulative stance toward this human gift. Lust is a sin, not because it is sexual, but because it exploits people. Instead of reverencing and celebrating the beauty and attractiveness of others, it turns them into objects.

Sexual fantasies become morally wrong when they reflect a persistent pattern of using people or violating relationships. Even though they are frequently spontaneous and involuntary, our sexual fantasies are important indicators of our sexual needs and interests. When there are consistent and recurrent cycles of exploitative or violent scenes, especially if these are dwelt upon and fostered by the individual, this is a sign of psychic, emotional, and spiritual illness.

Healthy sexual fantasies, on the other hand, are a normal and necessary part of psychosexual growth. They are not "impure thoughts." Rather, they are the creative way in which our imagination prepares us for mature love.

Phase II:

Psychosexual Preoccupation

"Teenagers are hormones with feet." This comment by an inner-city social worker was quoted recently in a national news magazine as part of a series of interviews exploring the sexual behavior of youth. Her comment probably flowed from years of practical experience — a kind of street-wise insight into the reality of the adolescent sexual response.

But her words also reflect a stereotypical view of this transitional time in our lives. Most of us can remember the familiar remarks about "growth spurts," "zits," and "raging hormones." As a young person, we may even have been the butt of these or similar comments. We may still be carrying some of the painful feelings that accompanied them.

There is a widespread tendency to see adolescent experience primarily in terms of biological and hormonal growth. As important as these physical changes are, the emotional and psychological factors have an even more profound impact. One of the predominant emotional patterns during adolescence is what we are calling "preoccupation."

First, a word about what we do *not* mean by this designation. We are not suggesting that teenagers spend most of their time thinking about sexuality. The operative word here is "preoccupation" — the intense personal concern that teenagers bring to all the changes going on within and around them.

This psychic attentiveness can take many different forms and expressions. Without pretending to develop an exhaustive list, we can safely say that as adolescents we were probably preoccupied with at least some the following issues.

Physical Changes and Personal Appearance

The experience of puberty varies greatly, both in terms of age and external characteristics. The normal onset of puberty, initiated by hormonal changes, can begin as early as eight or as late as fifteen or sixteen. The actual physical maturation can be completed within a year, or it can take more than six years. These variations are dependent on a multiplicity of factors, including heredity, nutrition, climate, and the percentage of body fat.

Our personal response to these changes also varies greatly. Some young people are excited about the prospect of puberty; others seem anxious or worried. Some appear indifferent; many simply take it in stride. No matter what form our outward presentation takes, most of us are inwardly sensitive to these physical changes. We instinctively know that this time of growth will determine our adult bodily appearance and the corresponding self-image that we will carry for our entire lives.

Understandably, our inner feelings may include a wide range of responses. We may be afraid that we are developing too soon, too late, too slowly, or too quickly in comparison to our peers. We might worry about our height, the contour of our body, the change of voice pitch, or the increased incidence of acne and pimples. We are distracted by our feelings. We develop "crushes" on classmates, teachers, counselors, or other adult mentors. We experience misunderstanding, abandonment, and rejection. We may be alternately excited or confused by our intensified sexual feelings and the physical responses that accompany them.

Our anxiety about this flood of change in our lives will sometimes be reflected in other forms of preoccupation — rapidly changing moods, a loss of interest in school, excessive daydreaming, and in some cases a drop in academic performance.

Peers and Social Pressure

As we begin to separate ourselves psychically from our parents or caretakers in our quest for personal identity, we often find ourselves in a dilemma. On the one hand, we want to assert our independence from the protection, the values, and the perceived limitations of our families. On the other hand, we are still wrestling with a deep need to belong. Most of us resolve this dilemma at this stage of our lives by trading in one form of dependency for another. At the same time that we push for more independence from our parents, we take the necessary steps to make sure that we "fit in" with our peers.

This need to be part of the group, to belong, is a powerful emotional preoccupation during our developing years. At times, it can be so strong that it becomes the emotional and ethical priority, the primary basis for decisions that range from the style of our clothes to the patterns of our sexual behavior. The adolescent who begins to notice, discuss, and engage in sexual activities, may be doing so, not because of a "hormonal push," but because of a "societal pull."

The Teen Subculture: Fashions, Fads, and Possessions

Young people (not to mention their adult counterparts) are strongly influenced by the rapidly changing consumer fads and social trends. In today's culture this includes the latest designer fashions, footwear, hairstyles, makeup, and MTV. It also extends to the preoccupation that teens have with personal possessions such as stereos, VCRs, TVs, personal computers, and other electronic equipment.

The concern with having one's own "things" is simply a reflection of the wider need that we have to develop our personal boundaries: to have our own room, to maintain a carefully guarded sense of privacy, and, of course, to have ready and confidential access to the phone.

Emerging Personal Identity

Beneath the variety of preoccupations that we have mentioned above, there is a deeper quest taking place in our lives. To our parents and teachers, we may appear to be moody, irresponsible, forgetful, and flighty. But beneath the outer turmoil and confusion, like a deep underground spring, there is a current of awareness, a flow of serious reflection going on.

As teenagers we are haunted by the same fundamental questions that generations of young people have had to confront. They are similar to the questions that Jesus must have wrestled with on his way to Jerusalem at the age of twelve. They are questions about the meaning and direction of our lives. Who am I? Who is the person beneath these conflicting needs and feelings? Will anyone find me attractive? Will I really be able to love someone? What am I going to do with my life? What should I study? What kind of a career should I pursue? What do I really believe about God and religion? What are my ethical values?

Viewed from the horizon of human history, these questions may not appear to be particularly significant. But when we are growing up, they are written in large letters on the pages of our hearts. They are the kinds of questions that we can answer only with our lives.

Phase III:

Relational Exploration

The desire to forge bonds of love begins at the moment of our birth and continues throughout our lives. In this sense, what we are describing as the third phase of adolescent psychosexual development — *relational exploration* — actually begins as early as the first experience of being nursed. It is developing when we begin to follow the eyes of our mother or play peek-a-boo with our father or other caretakers. We are pursuing the hunger for relationships when we feel threatened by the arrival of a new baby brother or sister, when we engage in sibling rivalry or play one parent off against the other in subconscious games of withholding or bestowing affection.

Young boys are growing in their bonding skills when they build tree houses or discover caves and form exclusive, tight-knit "boys only" clubs. Their passwords and stories, their fierce loyalty to one another, and their common "hatred" of girls is another important phase of exploring the mysterious world of "withness." Young girls frequently develop "best friends" — the classmate, cousin, neighbor, or fellow girl scout with whom they spend their time and share their secrets.

In the early stages of puberty there are dreamy-eyed looks, notes to be passed, telephone calls to make, pajama parties, lock-ins, and valentines. There are crushes, puppy-love, and posters of our favorite film and recording stars. Adults may smile condescendingly or be mildly irritated at these early forays into the world of romance, but they are necessary rehearsals for the real thing. For a young adolescent, the first stirrings of romantic interest and sexual desire are not something to be dismissed with adult cynicism; at that time in our lives, these are encounters with mystery and power. They are matters of emotional life and death.

Falling in Love

Somewhere in our adolescent years there is usually a relationship that takes us beyond the initial rush of feeling or earlier emotional crushes. This is no longer puppy love or mere flirtation. This is serious emotional business. We have fallen in love. Most likely it is not the Hollywood version complete with background music and stars in our eyes. But it is a serious and often shaking encounter with our selves and the power and presence of another person. It can be quiet and deep, or soaring and all consuming. It can be carried secretly in our hearts or spoken tentatively to the beloved.

Whatever its form or expression, this newer and deeper level of relating is more powerful and intense than before. It has far greater consequences and more emotional impact. We are standing now at the threshold of our adult lives. We are entering into relationships that may well give definition to the way in which we will express our sexual energy and engage in human intimacy for the rest of our lives.

Having said this, we must at the same time recognize that relationships at this stage of our development are still "exploratory." No matter what their intensity or their future direction, relationships at this point are still liminal and tentative.

This period in adolescence can be especially difficult for persons who recognize that they are attracted to members of the same sex. The "heterosexual assumption" of our culture confronts homosexual persons with painful choices. Either they must choose to disguise their orientation by dating persons of the opposite sex, or they must risk the rejection of family, friends, and classmates by being open about it. Many gay or lesbian adolescents find both sides of this dilemma to be unacceptable. In the end, they choose to withdraw socially until they graduate from high school and leave home.

Normal Narcissism

In our later adolescent years, most of us experienced a time when our psychic and emotional energies were focused on our introspective needs and personal concerns. This "normal narcissism" is a characteristic quality of our teenage years. There are exceptions of course, in that some young people achieve a level of emotional integration and the ability to be maturely other-centered rather early. For the most part, however, this phase of our development is characterized by a keen awareness of what "feels good" to us. We have become conscious of our uniqueness as emerging adults, the particular twists and turns of our personalities, the singular shape and form of our bodies, the excitement of our sexual response. As a result, we tend to be more focused on our needs, our emotional cycles, our interests and infatuations, our expectations, and our physical desires.

This normal narcissism is a step beyond some of the earlier forms of adolescent preoccupation that we discussed above. Its context is still the self and its needs, but its direction and energy are toward the other as fulfiller of these needs. We are "relational explorers" during this time of our lives, because we have not yet achieved the mature capacity for empathy and sensitivity to the inner world of another person. At this point, we are still exploring the other as provider of attention, comfort, pleasure, status, security, entertainment, and a host of other needs.

In essence this is a time of emotional and psychic convergence, perhaps even of conflict. Our newly emerging self-identity and self-awareness make us sensitive to our personal wants and needs. Our hunger to "connect" and to find a life partner propels those personal needs into dialogue with other people. If our psyches could break through the built-in emotional illusions at this time in our life and speak the truth, they might tell us frankly that they do indeed want it "both ways." They expect the ideal companion who is attractive *and* who also "adores" them — someone who is at once exciting and attentive to their every need and desire.

Levels of Physical Expression

In our culture, relational exploring among adolescents is frequently expressed, not only through the more traditional ways of hugging, kissing, and petting, but also through genital intercourse. *The Kinsey Institute New Report on Sex*(1990) reports that the age at which the average American first has sexual intercourse is sixteen or seventeen. Obviously, many experiment with this form of behavior at an even earlier age. By the time they are eighteen years old, 65 percent of boys and 51 percent of girls are sexually active. In the United States a teen gets pregnant every thirty seconds. And every thirteen seconds an American teen gets a sexually transmitted disease.

Statistics such as these can be used in many different ways. Some would refer to them as an indicator of the moral decadence of this culture and the need to return to stricter ethical values. Others point to this data as evidence that religious institutions and families have not done enough in the area of educating youth in sexual matters.

What seems to be missing in both sides of this debate is the attempt to address the issues that we are exploring here, namely, the dynamics of psychosexual growth that are taking place in young people at this age. What is missing is family and ecclesial formation regarding the *centrality of friendship* in human life. What is missing is a commitment to educate ourselves and our children in the *skills of human communication* — listening, attending, disclosing, and appropriate ways of dealing with conflict.

In our culture, and perhaps also in our churches, we consistently underestimate the ideals and values of young people. The majority of adolescents are not focused on attaining sexual gratification. Most young people instinctively sense that they are at a stage of relational exploration. Many simply want to engage in the search for authentic friendship. Unfortunately, in our society such a quest is often met with disbelief or even disdain. As a result, many young single persons find themselves in the dilemma of having to choose between temporary sexual relationships or emotional isolation.

"Be of love (a little) more careful than of anything." This line from an e. e. cummings poem could serve as a motto for our journey through adolescence. During our teenage years we learn that love is both a powerful energy and a fragile bond. We come to know its passion and its vulnerability. We realize that we need to be "care-full" of love, not because it is frightening, but because it requires deepening self-knowledge and reverence for others. Not least of all, we learn that, like the young carpenter from Nazareth, we need to grow in wisdom and grace.

QUESTIONS FOR REFLECTION AND SHARING

These questions have been designed to help you personalize what you have just read. They are a way of getting in touch with your own story, of exploring what in you needs further growth or healing. Do not feel that you have to respond to all of them. Also, you may wish to reflect on them over several occasions. You may find it helpful to spend some time in prayer with them, to record your responses in your journal, or in some cases to share your responses with a close friend or significant other.

1. What are your spontaneous memories of your adolescent years? Take some time to go back to your high school annuals or other memorabilia. What feelings and memories are evoked?

2. How did you obtain your first sexual information as an older child or a young adolescent? What were your parents' attitudes about sexuality? What messages did you get from them directly? Indirectly?

3. What are your memories around self-pleasuring during this period? What was your level of sexual exploration and experience? What kinds of feelings surrounded these experiences?

4. Were there any experiences of sexual trauma or sexual abuse during your adolescent years? If so, how have these events affected you? What kind of healing or help have you had as part of your recovery?

5. How did you feel about yourself as a young man or a young woman? What were your "self-messages" or "self-talk"? What was happening in your friendships and your relationships? Your dating history?

6. What awareness did you have about the direction of your sexual orientation? If you felt you were same-sex oriented, or wondered about this, how did you respond to this awareness?

7. Who were you able to talk to about sexuality as an adolescent? Who could you confide in? Get information from?

8. What do you recall about the content of your sexual fantasies during this time of your life?

9. What were your experiences of guilt during adolescence? What did you do with those feelings?

7

COMING INTO OUR OWN

Psychosexual Development in Adulthood

> The whole creation is on tiptoe to see the wonderful sight
> of the sons [and daughters] of God coming into their
> own.
> — Romans 8:19 (Phillips Trans.)

This past year we presented an adult education class on the topic of human sexuality at a local parish. During one of the discussion periods, a married woman in her late thirties shared the following observation: "This is the first time I've heard church professionals speak about the need for ongoing growth in intimacy. I've had the feeling that neither society nor the church understands how unfinished we are. They don't seem to take adult growth seriously."

Her comment provides a concrete starting point for our reflections on the adult stage of psychosexual development. Our experience indicates that there is a growing hunger for personal and interpersonal growth in our society. More and more people are "taking their adult growth seriously." They want to hone their communication skills and expand their capacity to be loving, compassionate persons. They are seeking ways of becoming more at home with their sexuality and deepening the quality of their relationships. Most importantly, they are envisioning maturity, not as a static reality, but as an unfolding journey.

101

What Is Maturity?

Most of us grew up with a rather narrow understanding of what it means to be an "adult." It was more of a cultural presumption than a philosophical theory, but it nevertheless influenced the way we understood ourselves and our lives.

The assumption went something like this. Sometime between the ages of fifteen and twenty-five, the physical, intellectual, emotional, and spiritual energies of our lives were expected to converge. At a certain critical point, *Voilà!* Off the human assembly line there came another "mature" human being. Of course, we weren't expected to be carbon copies of each other, nor were we "manufactured" with the same specifications. We came in a variety of models. Some of us were hard tops, others were convertibles. Some were straight stick, others were automatic. There was, however, one fundamental assumption regarding all makes and models: once you came off the assembly line, there were to be *no recalls*, just regular maintenance!

Obviously, this is an exaggeration, a caricature of how we actually viewed things. But there's a lot of truth here that resonates with most of us in our middle years or older. Early in our adult lives, we were expected to "have it all together" and get on with the business of living in a responsible fashion.

This perspective also applies to psychosexual maturity. By the time someone reached their mid-twenties they were expected to "settle down." This implied making a life choice regarding the manner in which they would express their sexuality: marriage, the single life, celibate or consecrated chastity. Finding a job, getting married, having children, and raising a family was the most common vocational pattern. In many religious traditions, there was a pragmatic stance toward the role of sexuality in marriage. The reproductive aspect was given clear priority over the interpersonal or "unitive" dimension of a relationship. If someone chose not to marry, there was an assumption that they would in effect become "asexual," or at least that the sexual interests and desires of their lives would be put "on hold."

In its early stages, the emerging science of psychology

tended to reinforce this static view of adulthood. Most behavioral scientists focused on childhood and adolescence as the primary means of understanding problems in adulthood. As useful as this perspective was, it inadvertently created the impression that development ceased at a certain point.

In the last several decades, this more static view of human maturity has undergone a significant change. Psychologists such as Carl Jung and Erik Erikson extended the notion of development beyond childhood and adolescence to encompass our entire lives. In recent years, further research and study has been devoted to adult life cycles and the rhythms of growth that continue until death.

The concept of ongoing development is not a twentieth-century discovery. It is as ancient as the biblical view of creation. In an earlier chapter, we noted the resonance between the new "cosmic story" that is emerging in our time and the dynamic view of creation and sexuality in the Hebrew scriptures.

In his view of the human person and the mystery of salvation, St. Paul reiterates the evolving, dynamic character of our lives. In his letter to the Romans, he uses the metaphor of "cosmic birth" as a way of describing our journey toward maturity: "From the beginning till now the entire creation, as we know, has been groaning in one great act of giving birth; and not only creation, but all of us who possess the first-fruits of the Spirit, we too groan inwardly as we wait for our bodies to be set free" (Rm 8:22–23).

From the perspective of Pauline spirituality "coming to birth" is a lifelong venture. In one way or another each of us continues to experience the "inward groaning" of coming to deeper maturity. We might encounter it when we confront our personal failures with courage and compassion, when we break through to greater self-knowledge or struggle with our fear of intimacy. We feel the groaning of birth at times of conflict with loved ones or when we are confused and discouraged about our apparent lack of sexual integration.

In Christian spirituality we are challenged to view these "birthpangs" from the horizon of hope. In the J. B. Phillips translation there is a striking image for this affirming vision: "The whole creation is on tiptoe to see the wonderful sight of

the sons [and daughters] of God *coming into their own*" (Rm
8:19, italics ours).

"Coming into our own" is another way of speaking about
our journey toward maturity. What implications does this have
for our psychosexual development as adults? Are there some
behavioral guidelines that will enable us to evaluate whether
or not we are "coming into our own" in our relational and
sexual lives?

In what follows we will attempt to answer some of these
practical questions. Following the "stage theory" of development that we outlined previously, we will discuss two phases
of adult psychosexual growth, namely *mutuality* and *ongoing
integration*. We will also explore some concrete indicators that
our readers might find useful in reflecting on their own level
of integration or personal maturity.

Phase I:

Psychosexual Mutuality

We have already spoken about narcissism as a dimension
of adolescent psychosexual development. This youthful self-
centeredness is a normal phase that we pass through in our
journey toward maturity.

But it is one thing to pass through this emotional phase; it
is quite another to settle in and spend the rest of our life there.
Ultimately, God has created us to move beyond our needs to
the concerns of others. Love is the reason for our existence,
the why of our being. To be is to be-with and to be-for.

Today most humanistic psychologists agree that the highest
form of self-actualization is expressed through our capacity to
care genuinely for other people. This echoes the gospel's call
to "lay down our lives" (Jn 15:13) in generative service of
others.

The first phase of adult psychosexual development —
what we are calling "mutuality" — is a way of describing
our maturing capacity to take up our lives with responsibility and to lay down our lives for others in shared love. It
is the transition from the adolescent focus on self to the
adult capacity for balance between self and others in our car-

ing. It is the ability both to give and to receive love in an enduring way.

Psychosexual mutuality is not limited to marriage or to a specific vocational path; it includes but is not limited to a sensitivity to another's needs in physical lovemaking. More inclusively, it is the ability to grow in authentic friendship, an inner stance of openness that all human persons are called to embrace, whether they are married, celibate, or single, whether they are heterosexual or homosexual in their orientation.

How can we tell if we are growing in the capacity and skills of mutuality? The following are some of the signs or characteristics of this phase in our adult development:

Accurate self-knowledge: When our self-perception is basically congruent with the way other people experience us. Without this capacity of self-awareness, we will not be conscious of how we "come across" to those we love and care for.

Empathy: The ability to have a "feeling connection" with others; to transcend our own needs and concerns so that we can be moved by the pain, the joy, the anger, or the fear of those around us, especially the significant others in our lives.

Interpersonal sensitivity: The capacity of being conscious and aware of the other person's needs. This is more than empathy; it includes intuitive and cognitive insight, as well as the willingness to respond to another person. With those with whom we have grown close, it involves the ability to *anticipate* their desires. If our state in life includes physical lovemaking as part of our relationship, interpersonal sensitivity also refers to the awareness and reverence that we have for each other's needs and preferences.

Trust: The foundation and primary building block for mutuality. Trust presupposes a capacity and a willingness to take risks, to surrender control over the beloved. It is the desire to validate the integrity of the other, even in the face of possible betrayal or rejection.

Equality: Another cornerstone for reciprocal love. If there is a real or perceived imbalance of power in a relationship, there cannot be authentic mutuality.

Capacity for self-disclosure: There cannot be mutuality without a shared experience of intimacy. The key to authentic intimacy is the ability and the skill with which we are able verbally to share our feelings and the world of our inner selves.

Spontaneity: The outcome or overflow of the above named qualities in a relationship. If two persons share a reasonable level of self-knowledge, empathy, sensitivity, trust, equality, and self-disclosure, there will automatically be an atmosphere of psychic and emotional safety — a setting in which playfulness, surprise, and wonder can flourish.

Phase II:

Ongoing Integration

Unlike the stages of childhood and adolescence, adult psychosexual development has only two phases or cycles. Essentially, this is because adult growth is open-ended and incomplete. As human persons we will always be, in some sense, unfinished.

With a reasonably healthy childhood and an adolescent environment that encourages our best efforts to grow, we can move into our adult years and achieve a level of mutuality in our relationships. Even if we have experienced the emotional setbacks that come from a dysfunctional family or the trauma of physical or sexual abuse, we can still come to a level of recovery and healing.

The Unfinished Journey

But no matter how gifted we are or how safe and validating our formative years have been, there is no magic moment at which we can proclaim to ourselves or to the world that we have "arrived." Similarly, no matter how much time and resources we have invested in the tasks of healing — whether in the form of personal reading and reflection, a Twelve-Step group process or other support group, spiritual direction, or intensive psychotherapy — there is no certificate of completion, no terminal degree for recovery.

In reality we are all "in recovery." None of us is exempt from the bruises and wounds of being human. We are all emotional wayfarers. None of us escapes the fears, the guilt, the mistakes, or the fallout of our brokenness. All of us stand in need of ongoing support and healing. We all have our loose ends, our unfinished business, our unresolved issues. "The price of wisdom," writes Robertson Davies, "is the loss of our innocence."

In the area of sexuality, ongoing integration may frequently take the form of doing "back-up" work in areas of our lives that were either skipped over, neglected, or simply not dealt with. There may be some days when we feel permanently fixated at some primordial form of immaturity. We feel uneasy with our bodies, disappointed with our ability to communicate, awkward at lovemaking, unable to communicate our feelings, overanxious about our health.

It may feel at times that we are regressing instead of progressing with our ability to relate to people. We may be embarrassed by the realization that we have been engaging in adolescent forms of behavior — flirting inappropriately, playing emotional games, crossing boundaries in expressing affection, becoming distracted or infatuated with someone at work, unfairly testing our beloved or our other friends, erupting in displays of jealousy or suspicion, pouting, withholding our caring, or giving someone the silent treatment.

Unless these behaviors form a persistent pattern, they are not irrevocable signs that we are twisted, inept human beings. More likely, they are simply reminders that we are still on the unmapped, sometimes confusing road toward human wholeness.

On the positive, hopeful side, ongoing integration is also a reminder that the horizons of growth are open-ended. We all share the capacity and the energy to keep on learning and discovering more about our bodies, ourselves, and the mystery of those whom we love. We are not only amazingly resilient, we are also remarkably resourceful. Pablo Casals, the world renowned cellist, was quoted at the age of ninety-one as saying: "It takes a long time to become young."

Psychosexual integration, therefore, involves a fluid and dynamic progression of growth along a wide continuum of behaviors and characteristics. It is reflected and expressed in all aspects of our lives, including the creativity with which we approach our work or ministry, the quality of our prayer and our play, the buoyancy with which we face adversity, and the life-enhancing nature of our relationships.

How can we know whether we are moving toward a reasonable level of psychosexual integration? Are there any concrete indicators that tell us we are on the right track? What are some of the signs that our relational journey is maturing in the graciousness of God's love?

We want to suggest some specific behavioral signs that point toward two different but related levels of psychosexual integration. The first of these levels is characterized by attitudes and patterns of living that reveal a basic and reasonable measure of relational maturity. The second level points toward deeper, more demanding dimension of growth and integration.

Level I: Basic Characteristics of Psychosexual Maturity

- Deepening personal awareness and good self-knowledge.

- Body comfort and a sense of being at home in our skin. Despite the exploitative propaganda of the media and advertising, we don't have to be young or have striking good looks to achieve a healthy sense of body image.

- Sustained and consistent involvement in close personal relationships and the capacity for intimacy. Such relationships are further characterized by:

  - honesty and trust

  - fidelity

  - awareness and openness about one's expectations

  - self-disclosure that is appropriate to the level of the relationship

  - open communication of feelings

  - physical expressiveness that fits with the level of commitment and closeness in the relationship

  - avoidance of control, manipulation, and abuse

- Faithfulness to primary commitments.

- Adequate knowledge of sexual anatomy and physiology, as well as current information on sexual issues and concerns.

- Comfort using sexual words and talking about sexual realities in appropriate settings.

- Not "overspiritualizing" sexual realities or engaging in emotional/psychic denial in relationship to them.

- Ability to make appropriate decisions and commitments involving sexuality.

- Taking responsibility for one's sexual expressions and behavior.

- Awareness of past hurts or traumas around sexuality and the willingness to take steps toward healing.

Level II: Signs of Deepening Psychosexual Integration

- A growing congruence between our personal behavior and our public, social commitments; a sense of integrity about our lives.

- The ability to name and articulate our sexual story in an appropriate setting (e.g., with a spouse, close friend, spiritual director, counselor, therapist, support group) and to understand how it has influenced our lives and relationships.

- A psychic and emotional *balance* between our sexual life and other aspects of living; neither being preoccupied with sexuality nor denying its place in our lives.

- Growing *integration* between the human and the holy, between our sexual energy and our spirituality. For example, when a married couple can experience as much closeness watching a sunset or praying together as they do sharing physical love.

- An attitude of compassion vs. self-righteousness in relationship to other people's sexual behavior.

- A deepening sense of *generativity*, i.e., the experiential knowledge that our presence to and with other people is life-giving and nurturing.

- Inclusivity in our relationships, whereby the beloved in our lives become companions in reaching out to a wider circle of persons without diminishing the depth of our primary commitments.

Psychosexual Integration and Genital Expressiveness

In past centuries, the church held up the state of consecrated virginity as a higher way of life than marriage. Recent church teaching has approached these two ways of life as different but equally valued means of living out the Christian call.

Ironically, in the aftermath of the "sexual revolution" and the human potential movement, many experts in the behavioral sciences are now beginning to pose a different question. Is it possible for someone to achieve psychosexual integration without engaging in genital expressiveness or physical intercourse? Many psychologists, pastoral theologians, and other helping professionals are quietly debating this issue.

Our conviction — which at this point is based more on the anecdotal experience of people than on formal research or theological tradition — is that while physical intercourse is certainly the more common form of human sexual expression, it is not in itself a *sine qua non* for arriving at psychosexual integration.

It is also our belief, however, that it is not possible to come to psychosexual maturity without life-giving *relationships*.

Some people choose a life of celibate or consecrated chastity because of a commitment to religious life or out of personal conviction. But there are many others who are celibate not by choice, but by circumstance. This group of people includes the separated and divorced, the widowed, some persons who are physically or emotionally handicapped, and those individuals who simply have not found a life partner. It seems presumptuous, if not arrogant, to assume that these individuals could not achieve a significant level of psychosexual integration.

In exploring this sensitive area, it is important to reiterate that we are speaking of sexuality in its more inclusive meaning as the other-orienting energy of our embodied existence. We understand sexuality as the primal force of interpersonal life, the God-created "allurement" at the heart of all human relationships. Depending on one's vocational path and commitments, this relational energy may or may not be expressed in a genital manner. In either case, it cannot find mature realization without authentic relationships. Without human intimacy we cannot become whole or holy.

The Sexual Revolution and Adult Development

We want to conclude this chapter with some reflections on current attitudes toward adult sexuality in our culture. The information explosion and the changing cultural mores in the post-war years, particularly in the mid-to-late 1950s, contributed significantly to the "sexual revolution" of the 1960s and 1970s. Despite its negative connotations, there were some positive results from this time of social upheaval. Several cultural stereotypes were challenged, including society's patriarchal bias, with its ethical double standard and its dominating attitude toward women.

But whatever else it accomplished, the sexual revolution did not necessarily enhance or deepen the quality of human relationships. Readily available information regarding sexual techniques and positions, does not, by itself, promote healthy, covenantal partnerships. Greater access to birth control methods does not automatically bring about stable marriages. Increased social freedom and greater explicitness in the media's treatment of sexual topics have not brought about a more mature generation of adults.

In an article entitled "A Revolution's Broken Promises," social commentator Peter Marin admits that even from the objective perspective of the behavioral sciences the upheaval in sexual mores has been at best ambivalent.[15] While looser restraints on sexual behavior create a climate of freedom and choice, this freedom is not unequivocally positive. The new spirit of openness can lead to emotional rejection, pressure, and conflict as easily as it can lead to personal fulfillment. For many people the pursuit of sexual satisfaction apart from the interpersonal values of human relationships has resulted not in greater "liberation," but in an encounter with personal bitterness and disillusionment.

Not surprisingly, the institution of marriage has not fared well during this time of social upheaval. The annual number of divorces has climbed steadily since the early 1960s and has leveled off only with the beginning of this decade. Occasionally, there are hopeful signs that people want to reclaim the value of healthy family relationships. At this point in our cultural history, we need to challenge ourselves to a vision that goes beyond safe sex. We probably don't need more information about sexual techniques and positions, but we do need more serious exploration into the interpersonal qualities that make for authentic intimacy and lasting commitment.

QUESTIONS FOR REFLECTION AND SHARING

These questions have been designed to help you personalize what you have just read. They are a way of getting in touch with your own story, of exploring what in you needs further growth or healing. Do not feel that you have to respond to all of them. Also, you may wish to reflect on them over several occasions. You may find it helpful to spend some time in prayer with them, to record your responses in your journal, or in some cases to share your responses with a close friend or significant other.

1. What have been your sexual experiences and behaviors as an adult? What do you feel best about? Worst about?

2. What are your most urgent questions? With whom have you shared them? How are you attempting to answer them?

3. What is the content of your sexual fantasy life at this time in your life? Are there any patterns that you recognize and tend to elicit of violence toward others? Manipulation? Self-depreciation?

4. How sensitive are you to the needs, moods, and desires of those closest to you? How do you express this sensitivity in words and actions?

5. How do you feel about your body today? How well do you know it? Care for it? What do you like best about it? What do you wish you could change?

6. How would people who know you best describe you? What adjectives would they use?

7. How faithful are you to your commitments? Can you trust others? Be trusted?

8. What needs to happen to promote greater growth toward wholeness in your relational/psychosexual life? What do you hope for the future?

8

SEASONS OF THE HEART

Adult Life Cycles and the Rhythms of Intimacy

> There is a season for everything,
> a time for every occupation under heaven.
>
> — Ecclesiastes 3:1

The author of the Book of Ecclesiastes is sometimes called the "existentialist" of the Hebrew scriptures. With poetic honesty, he unmasks our illusions about power, fame, and human achievement. He confronts us with our mortality and lays bare the fragile, often futile obsessions of our lives. He reveals the aching restlessness that stirs in our hearts and reminds us of the many ways we "chase after the wind" (1:14).

But Qoheleth (the "Preacher"), as the author of Ecclesiastes refers to himself, is not a nihilist. He is a believer who takes human life and its mysteries with utter seriousness. Even as he questions the transitory nature of all things, he celebrates the precious moments of beauty, the passion and warmth of human love, the quiet contentment of daily work, the simple joy of sharing food and drink with friends, the orderly sequence of the seasons.

Qoheleth stands in the "wisdom tradition" of the Hebrew people, a tradition that affirms human relationships as a precious gift of God. In contemporary language, we might describe him as an ancient psychologist of human development, an early explorer of what today we refer to as "adult life cycles." He is a mentor who leads us toward greater insight into the precious and precarious dance of intimacy. He invites us to reverence the underlying rhythms of our growth, to reclaim the mystery of our passage through time with those whom we love.

It is to these seasons of the heart in our adult lives that we now turn. Most of us can look back over our lives and see, if not a clear outline, at least a sense of rhythm and flow, perhaps even the hint of an unfolding pattern. It is possible for us to see our lives as graced and healed, as well as, at times, broken and wounded. We can recognize that there has indeed been "a season for everything...":

> A time for giving birth,
> a time for dying;
> A time for planting,
> a time for uprooting what has been planted...
> A time for tears,
> a time for laughter;
> A time for mourning,
> a time for dancing...
> A time for embracing,
> a time to refrain from embracing...
> A time for keeping silent,
> a time for speaking;
> A time for loving,
> a time for hating (Eccl 3:2–8).

Naming the Seasons of Our Lives

One of the tasks of ongoing psychosexual integration is the invitation to "name our days" (Ps 90:12), to reflect back on the story of our lives, and then to carry these memories with compassion and wisdom into the future. This chapter addresses this inner world of relationships: the soul's search for love, the ebb and flow of desire, the thrill of discovery, the agony of loss, the rekindling of dreams, the serenity of trust — the seasons of our hearts.

The framework that we have chosen to explore intimacy in our adult life cycles is simple and straightforward. We will reflect on the emotional and relational characteristics of three phases in our adult journey: early adulthood (approximately twenty to forty years of age), middle adulthood (approximately forty to sixty), and later adulthood (approximately sixty and after).

Our longing for closeness is an underlying need in each of these seasons of our lives. It is an integral part of the great questions of human living:

> The *identity* question: Who am I?
> The *intimacy* question: Whom shall I be with?
> The *life project* question: What shall I do?
> The *significance* question: What does it all mean?

Only a few generations ago, there was an expectation that by the time we were in our mid-to-late twenties we would have formulated our personal response to these questions. But the lengthening of the average life span, the insights of personal experience, and the contribution of developmental psychology have significantly altered that expectation.

Today we recognize that these questions are seldom answered in a definitive way at any single point in our lives. They recur in new circumstances; they resurface at times and in ways that we may not have anticipated. We may find ourselves wrestling with them at a crossroads in our career, when we are forced to reassess our vocational choices. It might be a time of conflict in our relationships when we struggle to reaffirm and deepen our earlier commitments. In some circumstances it may mean hearing these questions in an entirely new way and answering them by walking a different road altogether.

Early Adulthood
(Approximately Twenty–Forty)

In our contemporary culture, unlike most ancient societies, the initiation into adulthood is not a clearly delineated ritual or moment; it is rather a complex process or series of events that can be experienced and ritualized in a diversity of ways. For many of us it is symbolized by graduating from high school and turning our attention to the challenge of becoming personally and financially independent. For others it is the spiritual experience of validating our faith as a young adult Christian, celebrating one's Bar Mitzvah, or observing some other rite of religious transition.

These are symbolic transitions that bear strong cultural or religious implications. But there remains the practical process of "giving them flesh" — the challenge of implementing them in the theater of life.

A Time for Leaving

For most of us the entrance into adulthood becomes a psychic and emotional reality only when we physically leave home to pursue our own lives.

In today's stressful world, the process of leaving home is sometimes tentative and conditional. Many parents who thought they had successfully "launched" their children watch with concern and compassion as their offspring circle back to the nest to get financially refitted or emotionally refueled.

In reality, of course, we begin the psychic and emotional process of leaving home long before we load our personal belongings into the back seat of a car or rent a U-Haul truck to move out physically. This deeper journey of becoming our own person — what Jung refers to as the process of individuation — continues throughout our lives. In one sense, it is always "a time for leaving."

A Time for Choosing

No matter how differently we might actualize our coming of age, there are some underlying issues that we all share. The most obvious of these involves the far-reaching decisions we must make regarding our significant relationships and our life project: love and work, intimacy and productivity.

Whom shall I be with? In his theory of human development, Erik Erikson maintains that this is the central question of early adulthood. It implies the task of developing our capacity for authentic intimacy. We enter adulthood with many quiet — and often unspoken — questions about our relational lives. Who will share my life with me? With whom will I find love and mutual support? If I fall in love, will it last? If I feel called to a celibate way of life, with whom will I share intimacy?

What shall I do? In his groundbreaking study *The Seasons of a Man's Life*, Daniel Levinson speaks of this question as the task of "forming and living out the Dream." Clearly, he is referring to more than finding a job or settling for a career. This is an expansive question related to personal ideals and a life vision. What is my life's dream? How will my life make a difference? What are my gifts and how shall I express them?

In today's highly competitive society, these two decisions are often chronologically reversed: getting a job or starting a career frequently takes precedence over the relational needs of our lives. For most young adults the first and most urgent task is to prepare to make a living. They often have to balance their needs for intimacy and closeness with this more realistic demand on their time and energy. In the last three decades, this economic factor has been significant in raising the average age at which couples choose to get married. Males and females sometimes prioritize their "love and work" choices differently.

There is an additional form of discernment that homo-sexual persons usually have to face during early adulthood. They have to decide whether or when they will share the awareness of their sexual orientation with their family and friends. Despite many popular misconceptions, research continues to confirm that sexual orientation is not a matter of sexual preference, but something that we *discover* about ourselves, often quite early in our lives. In a culture that assumes that heterosexuality is normal, the decision to come out can be emotionally and psychologically stressful. In many circumstances, gay and lesbian persons still risk the rejection of their families, the loss of productive careers, and the judgmental attitudes of certain religious groups.

A Time for Risking

The centrality of personal decision and emerging responsibility is highlighted in our early twenties. As we stand at the threshold of adulthood we carry our dreams and hopes, our hunger for companionship and love, our desire to succeed and to achieve our goals. But we also carry our fears, our questions, and our silent apprehensions. During our youth there was time to linger with our daydreams, to image the perfect partner, to project our hopes on the wide screen of fantasy.

But now the time of daydreaming is past. In the mirror of life, our freedom stares back at us in the form of responsibility. Our fantasies are measured against real relationships. Our ideals are challenged to take on flesh and form. This is the time of resumés and interviews, apartment hunting, internships, and job performance reviews. This is the time of serious dating, of looking for someone who could be our life companion, the vertigo of falling in love. Or falling out of love.

Even if we choose to let this period of our lives be a time of hanging loose, we are still faced with familial and social pressures to make something of our lives — to define our goals and live a more purposeful life. However we choose to deal with these expectations, from a psychic and emotional perspective we will know what it feels like to be nomads and sojourners.

A Time for Embracing

Eventually we make the leap. After years of education and searching for the right position, we are hired. We launch out into our career. Likewise, after years of waiting and looking, we meet someone we really care for. We fall in love and move toward marriage or a covenantal commitment. Or after prayer and struggle, we choose the single life or follow the call of celibacy.

Whatever our choices, there is a common psychic element during young adulthood. Paraphrasing Qoheleth, we might describe it as a time of embracing — a season of intense involvement in life. We embrace a beloved in marriage, friendship, or a covenantal partnership. We embrace a career as a means of gaining financial success or personal fulfillment. We embrace a vision, a cause, or a conviction out of which we choose to live our lives. This is the *passionate* season — the time of "wholeheartedness," when we channel our physical strength, our psychic creativity, and our sexual energy into the pursuit of our goals.

In heterosexual relationships there is evidence that women

and men often enter into the relationship with different emotional expectations and needs. In the film *Sex, Lies, & Video Tape*, one of the female characters describes these differences in these words: "Men learn to love the person they're attracted to; women become more and more attracted to the person they love." Her comment may be an oversimplified summary of a more complex dynamic, but it captures some of the subtle variations in the way women and men express their sexual energy.

A Time to Refrain From Embracing

Not all relationships are healthy or able to withstand the inevitable forces of conflict. Love doesn't always move toward authentic intimacy. "Things fall apart," writes Yeats, "the center cannot hold." To meet with failure in love and intimacy is painful at any time in our lives. But during this period it is an especially devastating experience.

Whether or not we choose it, we are usually raw and emotionally vulnerable to the pain of misunderstanding, opposing needs, or betrayal. We tend to be passionate about everything, including the way in which we engage in conflict. Almost without warning, our wholeheartedness can plummet, like a skydiver without a chute, into brokenheartedness. Our passion for love collides head-on with the jagged edges of life. When marriages fail in the first decade or two, they are frequently contentious affairs with anguished endings and long, bitter aftermaths.

Middle Adulthood
(Approximately Forty–Sixty)

In his book *Modern Man in Search of a Soul*, Carl Jung observed that "we cannot live the afternoon of life according to the program of life's morning." For the past few decades the most familiar way of describing this shift in our personal priorities has been the popular phrase "midlife crisis." It is a term that is both helpful and unfortunate: helpful, because it invites us to be more attentive to the refocusing of psychic energy that takes place in our middle years; unfortunate, because it leaves us with the impression that this refocusing usually comes about abruptly through some form of emotional crisis. While this may be the case with some individuals, for many people it is a relatively quiet, far-reaching process. It would probably be more accurate to speak of a midlife transition — a journey toward a deeper dimension of the self.

What is involved in this transition? In particular, how does it affect our sexual energy and the patterns of intimacy?

In general, we can say that the first half of life — the morning — is primarily oriented toward relating to the outer world. It is concerned with establishing our ego-identity, our social roles, our place in the scheme of things. The second half of life — the afternoon — is oriented more toward the inner world. Without abandoning the outer world of roles and social tasks, it redirects our energies to issues of interiority, generativity, and intimacy. In the afternoon of life we are challenged to rediscover that we are human *beings* before we are human *doings*.

For our closest relationships this redirecting of energy can become an opportunity for growth in intimacy, or it can turn into an occasion for disillusionment and further withdrawal. In some cases it becomes a painful moment of truth that can even lead to the collapse of a relationship.

A Time for Reassessing

In one of his journals, Jean-Paul Sartre wrote that "by the time we are forty, we have our face." Whatever else he meant by this enigmatic phrase, he was clearly pointing to the ways that our past experience accumulates to shape our present stance before life.

By the time we are forty, we have a clearer sense of our gifts and limitations, both in terms of our career and our relational lives. By the time we are forty, we have come to some basic awareness about what we believe and value. We have probably had some mixture of success and failure in our life project. Along with our breakthroughs, we have also made our share of mistakes. Perhaps we need to re-examine our dream and our expectations.

We have also learned about the ecstasy and agony of love,

the ebb and flow of passion, the demands of parenting, the fragility of friendship, the loneliness and gift of celibacy. In our middle years we need to listen to our needs for intimacy with a new level of attentiveness.

This need to reassess our lives and relationships is one of the important tasks of midlife transition. It is a time to step back from our roles and return to the great questions. Is this what I want to do for the rest of my life? What options do I have? What is the quality of my relationships? What kinds of skills do I need to develop to grow in intimacy? Has my sexual expression of love become routine and lacking in meaning?

A Time for Trusting

During our middle years many of us face the realization that our earlier dreams for financial or vocational success will not be realized, at least not in the grand manner we might have anticipated. In turn, we may also have to become more real- istic about our level of physical energy, our eating habits, the amount of sleep we need, and the fact that our bodies are less resilient. We may recognize the need to move to deeper levels of intimacy, to be more compassionate with ourselves and our loved ones, to be more attentive to our changing emotions and moods, to be more reverent toward our bodies, to take more risks around self-disclosure, to ask for support and care from those we love.

What do all of these awarenesses have in common? They are quiet invitations to "come to terms" with the flow of time. This is a season of reconciling ourselves to life and to our relationships. This is not the same as giving up on life; rather it is a shift in what we most value in life. It is an act of hope, not an exercise in cynicism. It is way of redirecting our energy into deeper currents of life.

In this time of our lives, we are invited to be gentle with our limits, to come to grips with our mortality, to recognize that there are probably fewer tomorrows than yesterdays, to face the death of our parents, to share our fears of loss with those closest to our hearts.

A few years ago a married couple in their late forties asked us to work with them in therapy. We will call them Bob and

Sue. After the first few sessions, it became clear that this couple engaged in fighting to avoid deeper intimacy. They used
sarcasm to protect their vulnerability and their deeper feelings
of caring for each other. Ironically, their arguments functioned
as a means of having some contact with each other, while at
the same time providing enough distance to avoid the risks of
greater closeness.

This became particularly obvious one day when they re-
ported a bitter argument that had occurred the previous week.
For some time Sue had been asking Bob to increase the amount
of their life insurance coverage. His standard response was to
become defensive and angry, which in turn triggered a long
verbal battle. As they began to replay this argument during
the session, we asked each of them to stop for a moment and
become aware of what they were really feeling inside themselves. After a long silence, and with great difficulty, each of
them began to share their more vulnerable feelings.

With tears in her eyes, Sue spoke of her fear of losing Bob
through a heart attack — the way in which his father and two
uncles had died in their fifties. In turn, Bob shared his anxiety
regarding his family's health history, his inability to talk about
death, and his feelings of helplessness and guilt regarding the
life insurance.

This became a sacred moment for them, a time of mutual
compassion and understanding, a breakthrough to another
level of intimacy and love. They discovered that sharing their
genuine care for each other was a much more satisfying and en-
riching way of communicating than hiding their vulnerability
behind sarcasm.

A Time for Deepening

If we resist or reject the deepening process of midlife, our
lives will become increasingly empty and desperate. But if we
let go and move with trust into its deeper currents, this time
of transition can become a midlife *renaissance* — a rebirth of
energy, a growth in understanding, an appreciation for the
preciousness of life, a source of new creativity.

"My forties and fifties have been some of the best years of
my life." We have heard these or similar comments from peo-

ple who have discovered the richness of interpersonal growth in their middle years. They are feelings voiced by women who, after their childbearing years or following a divorce, experienced an awakening dream and followed it by returning to work, developing a new career, finding new relationships, or preparing for ministry. They are voiced by men who reassess the drivenness of their lives and choose growth in intimacy over career advancement. They are sentiments echoed by celibates — priests, sisters, brothers — who have developed deep friendships and find a new balance and satisfaction in their ministry.

"Generativity" is another word for this flowering of life from its depths. It is the deepening realization that we are more than our roles, more than our degrees and our bank accounts, more than our achievements or our failures, more than our productivity or our sales record, more than our marriages or our children, more than our vows or our ministerial positions, more than our sexual orientation or our gender. Generativity is the awareness that we are *life-giving persons* because of who we *are* and the authenticity with which we live our lives. It is the energizing presence that radiates from someone who has learned how to give and receive love.

Later Adulthood
(Sixty and After)

Our fascination with youth culture, body image, health consciousness, and independent lifestyles has combined to make the aging process for many people a dreaded and lonely experience. In contrast to earlier cultures where the elders were honored and respected, our society has come to view "getting old" as almost synonymous with being nonproductive, dependent, and marginalized. Instead of evoking the possibility of wisdom and accessibility, the aging experience tends to suggest images of Alzheimer's disease, nursing homes, and isolation.

There are signs of hope, however. As we move further away from cultural arrogance and narcissism, there are indications that we want to reclaim the value of compassion and respect for the inherent dignity of people. We seem to be becoming more attuned to family ties, friendship, tenderness, and honest affection.

This does not mean that we should over-romanticize the experience of aging. Ultimately, growing old is a pathway for the courageous, not the sentimental. In one way or another, it is a journey into frailty and deepening solitude. Like the coming of evening, it is enveloped by the mystery of death and the unknown. It moves inevitably toward physical pain, emotional darkness, and, for some, even the loss of the ability to communicate.

But in the face of frailty, aging offers its own encounter with love and intimacy. It can be a time of evening light and winter grace, an opportunity to grow still deeper in plumbing the depths of love, the quiet fire of passion, and the unfinished journey of self-revelation.

A Time for Holding

Ideally, our years of retirement should be a time of stepping back from the world of work and focusing on our network of relationships: our family, our spouse, our friends, our life partner. It should be a season for traveling and visiting, a time for gardening, reading, or pursuing the activities we didn't have time for when we were still working. There should be long, quiet afternoons with those we love, time to plant flowers and to pick them, warm celebrations and festive gatherings at holidays and anniversaries.

But even if the ideal does not hold true for us — if our health or our financial situation does not allow for these social activities — this is still a time for connecting and joining. It is the season for holding. It is a time for bringing life and people consciously into our hearts and reverencing them, a time of holding up our memories in gratitude, of holding on to hope and personal integrity, of holding out our hearts in welcome and accessibility.

It is also a time of physical holding and being held. In our culture, sexual expression is generally regarded as something for the young, the healthy, and the attractive. We tend to be uncomfortable thinking of an elderly couple engaging in sexual relations. Their psychosexual experience is often dismissed with statements like "they are too old for that." Despite these cultural stereotypes, however, the psychological need for intimacy and pleasure does not disappear in old age.

Whether or not we are married, we all need the physical presence of other people in our lives — the warm hug of a friend, someone to wipe our brow when we are sick, the reassuring touch of a family member when they are sitting beside us.

Even if a couple can no longer share physical intercourse, they can make love in other affirming and tender ways. At the end of a presentation we gave recently, a man in his late sixties was waiting near the speaker's platform in a wheel chair.

"Thank you for speaking of the importance of *touch* in relationships," he said. "Six years after my wife and I were married, I was in an automobile accident. Since then, I have been partially paralyzed and we have not been able to have sexual intercourse. But we have continued to make love through the gift of touch and by holding each other."

We all began our psychosexual journey as children through the gift of touch. In the evening of our lives, this mystery of holding and being held continues to nurture our bodies and our hearts.

A Time for Surrendering

One of the most prized qualities of adulthood is our sense of being in charge of our lives and our relationships. But this feeling of self-initiated power can easily deceive us. Even when we are at the peak of our health and creativity — presumably in our early or middle adult years — there is a certain illusion of control that is operative in our lives.

In her book *Necessary Losses*, Judith Viorst confronts this illusion and reminds us that "throughout our lives we grow by giving up."[16] Death will not be the first or only time that we have had to let go. If we have been open to life and its rhythms, we have been learning about letting go from the time we were very young. "Our losses include not only our separations and departures from those we love, but our conscious and unconscious losses of romantic dreams, impossible expectations, illusions of freedom and power, illusions of safety — and the loss of our own younger self, the self that thought it always would be unwrinkled and invulnerable and immortal."[17]

Later adulthood is an opportunity to name our losses, to choose freely to follow the flow of our lives. It is the season for *surrendering*, a time to let go of old hurts and feelings of bitterness. It is a time to free ourselves from the anger that has held us in bondage — anger toward our spouse or former lover, anger toward our children or our parents, anger toward the church or our religious community, anger toward ourselves and our personal limitations, anger toward God.

It is a time to let go of impossible dreams and regrets, to release ourselves from past guilt about sexuality and failed relationships. It is, in the end, a season of gentleness and compassion.

A Time for Communing

"In the evening of our lives," writes Augustine, "we will all be judged on love." Most of us come to an experiential sense of this truth long before we face God or judgment. Life has a way of revealing its own priorities. As we grow older, the essential values of life tend to stand out with greater clarity. The love of our friends, the closeness of family, the bonds of trust — it is to these realities that we look for consolation and hope.

Along with its many other manifestations, love usually looks for words. In every season of our lives, we rely on words to help us communicate what is on our minds and in our hearts.

In our later adult years, the gift of language continues to be an important vehicle in speaking our love. But there is another ability that begins to become operative as well. It is a like a language without words — a sense of presence that goes beyond geography, beyond physical presence, even beyond death. We give it many different names. We call it compassion, empathy, sixth sense, intuition, clairvoyance, contemplative awareness. In essence, it is love beyond words. *Cor ad cor loquitur*. Heart speaks to heart; deep calls out to deep. The sacramental word for it is "communion."

In the Apostles' Creed we proclaim our belief in "the Communion of Saints." From our human perspective this is an immensely reassuring vision. It confirms that the central mystery of our lives now and in heaven will be the same, namely, *to be in communion*. From the perspective of psychosexual development, this creedal statement radically affirms the dignity and goodness of human intimacy. It reminds us that love not only goes beyond words, but beyond death itself.

There is an old adage that reminds us that "you can't take it with you." It is, of course, referring to our worldly possessions. We will not take our house or our wardrobe into heaven. For that matter, neither will we take our outstanding bills or our unpaid mortgage.

But there are some things that we *will* take with us. We will carry with us the most essential dimensions of our human journeys: our values, our choices, and our relationships. We will take with us everything we know about love and intimacy, our attempts to integrate our sexual energy and to build mutuality, our growth in generativity and the ways that we have been life-giving persons. The liturgy for marriage puts it simply: "Love is our origin; love is our constant calling on earth; and love will be our fulfillment in heaven."

QUESTIONS FOR REFLECTION AND SHARING

These questions have been designed to help you personalize what you have just read. They are a way of getting in touch with your own story, of exploring what in you needs further growth or healing. Do not feel that you have to respond to all of them. Also, you may wish to reflect on them over several occasions. You may find it helpful to spend some time in prayer with them, to record your responses in your journal, or in some cases to share your responses with a close friend or significant other.

1. In one of his journals, the philosopher Søren Kierkegaard wrote that "we live our lives forward, but we understand them backward." Take some time in prayer or go for a long walk and look gently "backward" over your life, with a special focus on the "seasons of the heart." What "understanding" or wisdom around sexuality and love does your life story reveal? Can you put some of this into words? Share it with a trusted friend or spouse?

2. Take some time with the "Great Questions" (Who am I? Whom shall I be with? What shall I do? What does it all mean?). How has your response to these fundamental questions in your life changed or developed over the years? What meaning or importance do you see in these changes?

3. What images and feelings does the phrase "leaving home" evoke in you? Take some time to reflect on the phases or stages of this process of leave-taking in your life. Is there a part of this journey that is unfinished for you?

4. Do you prefer to speak of "midlife crisis" or "midlife transition"? Why or why not? What have been the major shifts in your relational and psychosexual story during your middle years?

5. Judith Viorst speaks of the human challenge of coming to grips with the "necessary losses" in our lives — those inevitable experiences of letting go that all of us must face. What about the *unnecessary* losses" — those unexpected, early, devastating encounters with accidents, brokenness, illness, or death? How have you responded to them? What effect have they had on your relationships and ability to love?

9

TO BIND UP HEARTS
THAT ARE BROKEN

The Wounds of Psychosexual Development

The Spirit of the Lord Yahweh has been given to me,
    for Yahweh has anointed me.
He has sent me to bring good news to the poor,
   to bind up hearts that are broken;
   to proclaim liberty to captives,
    freedom to those in prison;
to proclaim a year of favor from Yahweh,
   a day of vengeance for our God,
to comfort all those who mourn and to give them
    for ashes a garland;
   for mourning robe the oil of gladness
for despondency, praise.

                 — Isaiah 61:1–3

The evangelist placed these words of Isaiah on the lips of Jesus as he began his public ministry. Luke deliberately positions the carpenter from Nazareth in the synagogue, unrolling the scroll of the prophet Isaiah, searching for his message of consolation. From the outset, Luke wants to present Jesus as the one who understands and reaches out to hearts that are broken. As his ministry unfolds, the words of Isaiah are fulfilled as the brokenhearted find healing in Jesus.

In the synagogue and private homes, in the towns and the countryside, on the sabbath and on ordinary days, he meets them. They are the infirm, broken, despondent people. Sometimes one by one, other times in crowds, during the day and even by night, they come to him. Strangers. Relatives. The wealthy. The poor. A father pleading for his little boy, caught in the grip of a mysterious malady. A little girl nearly drained of life. A leper. A woman lost in the crowd who wants only to touch his garment. Wherever they find him, he receives them. Whatever the repugnance of their ailment, they are welcomed by this man who seems to find no one, not even the sinners, too objectionable to touch or too debilitated to experience healing.

The range of human suffering that Jesus encountered was described according to the mentality of the day. For example, psychological disorders were often interpreted as demonic possession. Since the science of psychology had not yet been born, the people had no other framework within which to understand the many troubling conditions and alienating behaviors they experienced in certain individuals.

In Jesus' day, a man who did not talk could be identified as a "dumb demoniac" (Mt 9:32). Today, that man might more accurately be diagnosed with a psychological condition that has left him unable to communicate effectively. Whether his suffering is attributed to demonic possession or to a psychological illness, one thing is certain. The inability to communicate is heartbreaking.

What does this have to do with sexuality? How do the words of Isaiah relate to the problems we encounter with psychosexual development? More specifically, how can someone who dealt with lepers and demons be an occasion for hope for a person whose life has been bruised by psychosexual trauma? Ultimately, our growth is directed toward the adult capacity to form and sustain life-enhancing relationships. It is pointed toward love. It has to do with the stuff of the heart. When psychosexual development does not unfold in a healthy way, our relationships are adversely affected. When normal psychosexual development is severely thwarted or even destroyed, nothing can break hearts quite so tragically.

The significance of the gospel healing stories does not reside in the specific types of ailments Jesus cured. Nor do these stories speak to us only insofar as we can match our diseases to theirs. It is precisely their ability to transcend medical diagnosis and the limits of time that enables them to be good news for us today. They are our stories. Jesus is our healer. The power of the scriptures to give us images for our own healing is not limited by the name of our pain. When prayed with the eyes of faith, the message of Isaiah is a promise for our own troubled lives and broken hearts.

In discussing the stages of psychosexual development from prenatal life through adulthood, we have looked at how we move toward integration when conditions are favorable. While ideals are important, realistically we rarely have the optimum conditions that enable our psychosexuality to unfold smoothly and painlessly. Rather, we encounter obstacles, whether due to the limitations of our parents and caretakers, the ordinary human failure in ourselves and others, or the inevitable losses and disappointments of life. Sometimes our hearts get broken before they are even old enough for mature love.

The paradox of psychosexual development lies in the fact that we are at once fragile and resilient. Our developing psychosexuality is capable both of being wounded and of being healed. It can be as familiar with tragedy as it is with triumph. In fact, a central aspect of psychosexual integration in our adult years involves tending its wounds.

In this chapter, we want to look at some of the things that can hinder the process of healthy psychosexual integration. What are the causes of psychosexual injury? More important, how does it affect the adult capacity for mutuality and intimacy when our hearts get broken early?

The Spectrum of Psychosexual Wounds

Most of us carry some regrets about our psychosexual past and can identify limitations in the way our development unfolded. But there are degrees of damage that can be sustained. Some problems are temporary and may be easily remedied when we have new, healthier experiences or are graced with a healing relationship. Others are so devastating they create permanent damage and have lifelong consequences.

In addition, some psychosexual events are always hurtful, while the consequences of others depend more on the situation. For example, sexual abuse is universally destructive, regardless of age, frequency, or nature of the abuse.

The effects and long-term consequences of other psychosexual experiences depend on the personality of the individual, and the circumstances in the environment. For example, medical examination of the genitalia, being discovered during normal childhood sex play, punishment for using sexually explicit words, and other embarrassing or punitive experiences may have varying effects on different children. The impact may be greater on individuals who are particularly sensitive, who have been previously traumatized, or whose tendency to internalize and personalize the negative consequences of events is greater than average.

For example, nine-year-old twins, Mark and Andrew, accidently find a hard-core pornographic magazine while playing in the basement. Their mutual curiosity prompts them to page through it. Discovered by their father, the boys are harshly spanked. Mark attributes this treatment to his father's quick temper and does not believe that he did anything wrong in checking out a magazine that he quickly decided was "pretty disgusting." Later, Mark tells his best friend what happened, and the two boys agree that the spanking was unfair.

Andrew, on the other hand, broods and remains hurt and embarrassed. He discusses the event with no one, not even Mark. The more he thinks about it, the more he feels like a bad person inside. He attributes the punishment, not to limitations within his father, but to some reservoir of "badness" within himself. Obviously, Andrew's tendency to internalize painful events and to blame himself for causing them may make the impact of this psychosexual punishment more damaging for him than for his twin brother. In a very real sense, some of his healthy freedom to explore sexuality has been damaged. Shame and anxiety about sexuality have begun to bruise his heart.

Psychosexual Wounds: Led Away From Intimacy

When something happens to wound our psychosexual development, our emotional maturation can remain in a fixed position. Our bodies will continue to grow and develop, hormones will surge at the appropriate time, and the secondary sex characteristics of adolescence will appear. We can even marry and have children, all the while being psychologically detained at a much younger stage of development. When this happens, a host of unpleasant and even harmful consequences may befall our relationships. We can, quite literally, be led away from love.

Psychosexual fixation is similar to being trapped in a maze or caught in a holding pattern. We struggle. We worry. We are preoccupied with ourselves. We have needs that are unfocused or feel too big to meet. No matter how hard we try, our relationships seem to go nowhere. Ultimately, our ability to engage in mutual, self-disclosive, adult friendship is at stake as we move through the process of psychosexual integration. Anything that damages the process has a corresponding effect on our ability to love.

Less extreme and perhaps more common than true sexual fixations are developmental delays or temporary setbacks. These can occur when there are gaps in the area of our psychosexual integration. Instead of being irrevocably stuck, we are simply slowed down. We experience incompleteness in our psychosexual wholeness.

Whether held captive in the prison of a damaged psychosexuality or simply detained along the way toward integration, we feel shackled. Like the captives of Isaiah (61:1), we yearn for release. The Hebrew word for "captive" refers to those who have been physically captured and taken away to a place of confinement. For Jesus, it meant anyone who was oppressed, any person whose freedom to be fully whole had been taken away. It meant the blind man and the bleeding woman. It meant the outcast and the poor. It means you. It means me. It means all of us who struggle to be released from whatever binds our capacity to love well.

The Many Sides of Psychosexual Bondage

We can be taken captive in a variety of ways. Some prisons surround our bodies with steel bars. Others erect a cage around our souls. Either way, our movement is restricted and fear is our constant companion.

Imprisonment is an apt image for those who have experienced psychosexual trauma. Even those whose journey toward integration has been only slightly injured or delayed will speak of being trapped in discomforts and confined by the tightness they feel around their sexuality. Whenever healthy growth is oppressed, we — like Isaiah's captives — can be led away in bondage.

It is ironic that popular understanding equates bondage with attaining sexual pleasure in the context of being tied up — something most persons regard as sick or perverse. This is not how we are using the term. Since bondage involves a lack of freedom in some part of the total self, any form of it leads us away from love.

Bondage, then, in the biblical sense, describes the imprisonment of our psychosexual energy. The term can apply to anything that "ties up" our freedom, limits our self-awareness, restricts our capacity for self-disclosure, or reduces our sense of personal responsibility for our own sexual choices and behaviors. Anything that causes us to associate our sexuality with shame, fear, harm, anxiety, anger, physical pain, unhealthy guilt, failure, incompetency, or violence can lock up our sexual energy. This will, in turn, inhibit our normal growth to some degree. Some of the more common sources of psychosexual imprisonment include: (1) *trauma*, (2) *punishment*, (3) *unhealthy guilt*, (4) *failure*, and (5) *narcissistic indulgence*.

Although these can occur at any age or stage of development, our formative years are perhaps more vulnerable to their influence. The earlier these experiences, the more they impair the foundation of future growth. When problems occur later in the developmental cycle, particularly if maturation to that point has been healthy, at least we have a core of psychosexual strength on which to rely.

Trauma: Assault on the Soul

Sexual trauma is more than a violation of the body; it is an assault on the soul. It sears the core of a person. It can carry the personality into bondage and break the heart.

Any psychosexual event that evokes feelings of embarrassment, anger, or pain may traumatize us to some degree. In particular, whenever sexual realities become fused with shame the potential for damaging our sexuality is great. The following is a partial listing of experiences that can serve as sources of psychosexual trauma:

- Sexual, physical, or emotional abuse

- Medical examinations and procedures involving the genitals, anus, or breasts

- Discovery during normal childhood sex play

- Frequent enemas or rectal temperature checks

- Exposure of the genitals, breasts, or buttocks

- Frequent or harsh spankings

- Failure to receive accurate and age-appropriate sex information and education

- Being the recipient of a sexually transmitted disease

- Concern, confusion, and pain regarding sexual orientation

- Sexual harassment, psychosexual ridicule

- Being the victim of sexual malpractice (i.e., having sexual contact with one's therapist, doctor, confessor, academic professor, minister, or other helping professional)

Sexual abuse is the most devastating source of psychosexual trauma. Regardless of whether it involves penetration of bodily orifices or gentle tactile fondling, whether it occurs a single time or repeatedly over many years, whether the victim fights or submits, whether the perpetrator is known to the victim or is a stranger, sexual abuse always leaves scars. The circumstances may vary greatly, but no one emerges from sexual abuse unscathed. No matter how much interior strength a person may have, how much conscious awareness of the assault, or how much he or she may want to believe that "it didn't really affect me all that much," harm has been done and needs to be addressed. Sexual abuse may be one area where the old adage "Time heals all wounds," is farthest from the truth. Neither the passage of time nor increasing emotional distance from the event automatically heals the damage perpetrated by sexual abuse.

For our readers who have survived this assault on the soul but have never worked through the trauma in therapy, we would like to encourage you to give yourself this opportunity for greater healing.

Not all sources of sexual trauma are the direct result of an abuser. Some are the unfortunate byproduct of illness, injury, or accident. Still others occur because someone is careless, ignorant, or makes an honest mistake. In looking back over our sexual stories, we can often tell if there is some lingering discomfort that haunts our memory. Perhaps it was standing naked in the shower room after a ball game with our eighth grade classmates and being taunted because ours was the only body that was still undeveloped. Perhaps it was surgery for a bladder problem when we were old enough to be mortally embarrassed by the catheters and examinations. Maybe it was the gradual recognition during our teenage years that we were homosexual, accompanied by the lonely awareness that there was no one with whom we could share this information or process its meaning for our lives.

We all have a category for sexually embarrassing moments in our psychosexual sexual stories. Sadly, some of us also have a category for "sexual traumas I have known." Sharing the little ones, the safer ones, with a close friend or significant other can often help relieve some of the discomfort. It can feel as though we are loosening some of the bonds that keep us tied to the prison of shame.

Punishment: Sexuality Out of Favor

It is a great gift to be given the assurance that our sexuality is good, that it is not only an acceptable part of us, but a graced part as well. We all need to know that our sexuality is, at its core, in favor.

In addition to the many forms of trauma, punishment can also cause our psychosexual development to become stalled or even arrested. It can turn the gift of sexuality into an unbearable burden. Punishment can make our relational energies and affectional interests feel out of favor. In the biblical sense, when something is out of favor, it is no longer a source of life.

When Isaiah looks forward to "a year of favor from Yahweh" (Is 61:2), he uses a Jewish phrase associated with Jubilee, whereby the forgiveness of debts, the release of slaves, and the offer of mercy were held up as ideals among the Jews. The Hebrew word "favor" means "to give pleasure." Isaiah 61 is steeped in Jubilee language. He looks forward to a time when mercy, compassion, and forgiveness will replace the oppression and unjust imprisonment of God's people. He promises that one day the people will be "pleasured" with freedom and surprised with liberation. Jesus of Nazareth carries Isaiah's hope forward in time.

At its best, our sexuality, along with other dimensions of our humanness, ought to be a source of pleasure for us. It ought to liberate us for relationships and free us to love. But it can do that only when it is free itself. A sexuality that has been fettered by oppression or imprisoned by harsh punishment can hardly be a source of relational liberation.

Punishment can cause damage to our psychosexual development whenever it is harsh, inappropriate, confusing, or shame inducing. When it includes public humiliation, the damage can be that much greater. Punishment is equally tragic if it causes us to feel that our sexuality is bad, dirty, naughty, or less noble than other aspects of our humanity.

When we were children, we might have been punished for fondling our genitals, using sexually explicit words, engaging in childhood sex play, or being curious about sexual matters. Punishment can begin as early as infancy.

Joe is a married deacon who has had a lifelong problem with compulsive masturbation. Recently, his older sister told him of a memory she had of his infancy that had troubled her for many years. "You were about four or five months old, and I was changing your diapers. I was about nine. Suddenly, mother came into the room and began to scream that I shouldn't let you touch yourself. She roughly grabbed your hands away from your diaper area and slapped them. You started to cry. She kept yelling 'dirty' and 'naughty.' I know she did that more than once. I've sometimes wondered if it affected you."

This kind of punitive behavior can indeed affect us. First, Joe's natural need to explore all parts of his body was thwarted, creating anxiety. Since other forms of body touch were allowed, the anxiety probably focused around his genitals. Second, as he heard the scolding words, issued simultaneously with his hand-genital contact, he may have experienced that genital touch brought both pleasure and punishment. This kind of conflict is sometimes associated with the development of repetition compulsion — the need to continually (compulsively) repeat an act in order to resolve the anxiety and ambiguity associated with it.

While most of us were not victims of such severe punishment, we might have been scolded or embarrassed in other ways. Sometimes, talking about early memories with someone else who was there, and may remember more than we do, can give us greater insight around our current psychosexual issues. It can lead us out of the confinement of unknowing and into the light of understanding.

During the next phase of childhood psychosexual development (sexual awakening), we became more obviously sexual. Some of our parents may have felt uneasy with our increasing sexual interest. Depending on their levels of body comfort, they may or may not have tried to discourage our toddler efforts to become more familiar with our bodies.

There is a major difference between teaching healthy sexual discipline and inflicting punishment. We were disciplined in helpful ways when our parents gently explained to us that our genitals are special parts of our bodies and need to be covered. Teaching us proper sexual conduct was most helpful to us if it began during sexual awakening, when other forms of discipline were also being initiated.

During the final phase of childhood — psychosexual socialization — punishment most commonly occurs in response to childhood sex play or sexual behaviors that are considered inappropriate in public for an older child.

Sometime before puberty we became capable of comprehending right and wrong. This time of moral awakening has traditionally been called the age of reason. It coincided with the time in our life when we became capable of making informed choices, thinking about alternatives, and being aware of consequences of our behaviors.

During this developmental period responsibility for sexual behaviors assumes more prominence. Before the age of five or six, our sexual behaviors were governed primarily by drives, instincts, and curiosities. Even though we were capable of naughty behavior, we did not engage in sexual sin. Some aspects of our sexual behavior might have been socially inappropriate or mischievous. However, we did not have sufficient cognitive development to make decisions involving both intentionality and informed consent.

Ellen is a twenty-seven-year-old woman who has a memory that illustrates the life-giving effects of open communication between parents and children around sexual matters during this phase of development. It also reveals the important difference in outcome between providing discipline and inflicting punishment:

I was about ten years old and my best friend, Louise, and I were in the garage playing "doctor." She was lying on an old chaise lounge and I was "examining" her by looking inside her panties. My father came in to get some tools and surprised all three of us! I was so embarrassed but dad was great. He just said, "Excuse me girls, I didn't mean to intrude." Later that night, when we were alone in the living room, Dad told me that he was sorry if he embarrassed us. We had a wonderful talk then about how it was normal to be curious about sex and that the most important part of it was love. Dad's respect for my childhood sex play experience taught me the most important sexual lesson of my life — that sex involves reverence for myself and others. It's one of the most treasured memories of my life and a sexual lesson I have never forgotten.

Adolescence. That time for growing in wisdom and grace. What do you remember from those awkward, gangly years about the ways in which you were disciplined — or punished — for your sexual interests and behaviors? Were there dialogues or shouting matches? Was there heavy silence or open conversation? Did your desire to connect meet with advice, dogmatic orders, threats of sexual sin, or with discussions about how to develop healthy and responsible relationships? Did your sexual energy find favor during your teenage years, or did it enter bondage? Did your heart get broken by a first love gone awry?

Some of us may have emerged from adolescence suffering from punishments inflicted not by our parents, but by our fellow teens. Others may have experienced punitive responses from relationships even later, during our adult years. Such punishments can be as subtle as they are destructive:

- Sue's boyfriend dumped her when she told him she was not willing to have sex with him.

- Don became angry that Doris dated other boys besides him, so he spread it around school that she was "an easy make."

- Mike was shunned and talked about behind his back because his classmates thought he was gay.

Psychosexual punishment can occur at any age. It can be as direct as a slap on the hand or as covert as the cold shoulder treatment. Either way, it hurts. It produces shame. It can cause our sexual energy to lose connection with its source — the great cosmic fire — and the God who is its author.

Guilt: Putting On a Mourning Robe

Guilt. It is that familiar feeling of heaviness that washes over us when we have done something wrong. Guilt involves mourning the loss of our innocence. Healthy guilt, feeling bad when we have hurt someone or violated our standards, is a necessary component of psychological health. Healthy guilt acts as a kind of inner voice, calling forth awareness between right and wrong, prompting us to cease harmful behavior and make amends for any wrongs committed. Guilt is apt to be healthy when it is proportionate to the wrong that we have done.

There are some persons who are incapable of feeling guilt, even when they have caused great pain to others. The inability to feel appropriate guilt is one of the symptoms of a psychiatric condition known as Antisocial Personality Disorder. Persons who merit this diagnosis are typically very self-centered and are not at all bothered if they hurt or use people. Often times, people who sexually abuse others fall into this category.

At the other extreme, we have persons who feel guilty when they shouldn't. They range from the individual who feels guilt that is disproportionately large in relationship to a minor fault or innocent mistake to the person who is enveloped in remorse, even in the absence of any wrongdoing. Such individuals often suffer tormenting anxiety about their perceived sinfulness. Sometimes referred to as scrupulous, they continually ruminate about past failures. Occasionally called the Catholic Disease in the psychiatric literature, scrupulosity has been prevalent among those who interpreted the codes of their religious faith with rigidity or unusual intensity.

Unhealthy guilt can damage our psychosexuality. Many Catholics who grew up before the Second Vatican Council learned to associate sinfulness with any deliberate sexual thought, feeling, or activity that was not confined to marriage. For those who still carry guilt in relationship to the normal processes of psychosexual development, contact with a spiritual director or understanding minister can help replace unhealthy guilt with compassion. When scrupulosity is a problem, this is considered a psychiatric condition, not a religious issue, and requires the attention of a competent therapist.

Failure: The Road to Youthful Despondency

"I was so excited about the prom. When I finally got the nerve to ask Sharon, she told me she was already going with another guy. Two other girls turned me down. After that, I was too devastated to ask anyone else. At sixteen, I felt like a social failure."

"Whenever I think about high school, I get a knot in my stomach. I was painfully self-conscious. Every time I opened my mouth I said the wrong thing. I was never part of a crowd. God, it was lonely."

Ashes. Despondency. Mourning robes. The images in Isaiah's fourth Servant Song can aptly describe our experience when we encounter relational defeat. Several things can happen when we find ourselves wandering in the ruins of our foiled attempts to personalize our psychosexual energies. We can despair of the possibility of finding friendship and turn away from it altogether. Or we can exchange the dreams of friendship for the quick comfort of sex-only relationships. If we lack sufficient communication skill and self-confidence to experience success in true relational exploration, at least we can have physical closeness — for a while.

When we fail in our early attempts to form romantic friendships, the substitution of genitality for relationality can seem like the next best choice to some. In a culture where the role models for romantic love are too often soap opera couples and video stars, serious effort to form friendships can be bypassed in favor of casual sexual liaisons.

Although church teaching forbids it, it must be acknowledged that many young people today engage in genital experience long before marriage. Even aside from the moral questions, there are long-term relational effects from these early genital experiences. Like many other firsts in our lives, one's first sexual sharing sets the stage for all subsequent ones. It becomes a reference point in the psyche for future genital relationships. Out of it are born the expectations, anticipations, feelings of personal worth, and sense of competency that will subconsciously be attached to sexual experiences to come. If the first one feels like a failure, either in terms of the setting, the partner, or the actual experience, that sense of disappointment will be brought forward.

For example, if one's first sexual intercourse takes place in hurried anxiety, with a partner who has no commitment to the relationship, then the aura surrounding that event will intrude like an uninvited guest into one's next sexual experience.

Conversely, when commitment, fidelity, trust, love, and emotional sharing form the context of one's initial sexual experience, all of that becomes the background music for tomorrow's love.

Our early experiences with friendship formation and/or sexual experience might not have provided the inspiration for a love song. Sometimes, our disappointments and failures can be the learning ground for fine tuning our relational skills or rethinking our values. Other times, particularly when failure becomes a pattern as opposed to an occasional experience, isolation, superficiality, and despondency can become all too real.

Whenever we encounter failure in our relationships, we need to allow ourselves to feel the loss, think about its causes, and experience mourning as a part of our healing. If we are to exchange "ashes for a garland" (Is 61:3), we must first embrace the ashes.

Narcissistic Indulgence: A Garland Without Ashes

We said earlier that self-preoccupation is a normal though temporary phase of adolescent psychosexual development. If as children and teenagers we got the message that "the world was our oyster" and it could stay that way forever, we might have been the unfortunate victims of the abuse of indulgence.

Narcissistic indulgence occurs when we are protected from pain, shielded from facing the consequences of our behavior, and given the message that we are not just special, but superior to almost everyone else. If we were given an overabundance of attention, protection, material goods, or favored treatment, our ability to empathize and place the concerns of others on an equal par with our own could have been damaged. There is corresponding damage to our ability to enter into relationships where mutuality and interpersonal sensitivity make intimacy possible.

Perhaps the greatest tragedy for the middle-aged narcissist is that he or she lacks the interior capacity to maintain the one thing that is so strongly desired — the experience of being truly special to a significant other. Lacking both accurate self-knowledge and an ability to admit mistakes, the person with a narcissistic personality has great difficulty with genuine self-disclosure. When anyone displeases a narcissistic person or fails to measure up to that person's expectations for almost constant adulation, the relationship often ends. All of these

qualities limit the depth of relationships, keep sharing superficial, and make permanency difficult. Because the narcissistic
person is oriented toward personal pleasure, the slow give-
and-take of ordinary human struggles to achieve and maintain
closeness is not tolerated well. Having little patience for working out long-term commitments with their ups and downs,
the narcissistic person often exchanges the possibility of real
intimacy for superficial genital sharing.

Isaiah's words anticipate a day when captives are liberated
and mourners will be comforted. They also remind us that
there are many ways to be taken captive and many sides to sadness. The self-centered person is a prisoner of indulgence. He
or she is mourning the loss of the real self — the best, truest
self, the self that has the capacity for mature love. The message
of Isaiah carries still another, more poignant truth. The "oil
of gladness" does not come without cost. It is often wrapped
in a mourning robe. A garland is all the more beautiful, not
when it substitutes for ashes, but when it follows them.

The Long-term Effects of
Early Psychosexual Wounds

Whenever the losses, wounds, and brokenhearted memories
of our early psychosexual histories outweigh the recoveries
and promises of the future, the effect can be no less than
lifelong difficulty giving and receiving love. The outline at
the end of this chapter summarizes some of the effects of
psychosexual damage. It identifies some of the characteristics
of adults whose relational capacities are impaired. In reading
the outline, it is important to keep in mind the caution from
an earlier chapter: If you see hints of yourself in some of the
characteristics, "don't judge it or you will bruise it."

While the words of Isaiah assure us of God's concern for
our broken hearts, simply hearing these biblical phrases does
not automatically effect healing. The consoling message of
scripture cannot be equated with a magical formula for recovery. Rather, it is an announcement of possibility for all the
oppressed and unfree places in our lives. When we pray these
words and personalize them, we can find a starting place for
our healing. When we trust that growth in psychosexual inte-

gration is possible for us, then the hard work begins. We have to set out, as Jesus did, to the highways and hillsides where our sores keep us on the fringes of friendship or hidden in tombs.

This involves looking over our lives, the history of our loving, and telling our sexual story with the candor of the woman at the well. We must tell it first to ourselves and then to someone who will understand and help us name its truth more clearly and see its power to transform us. It means identifying the places in our lives where integration is missing or where more growth is possible.

Like the woman with the lost drachma, it means naming what is gone — or out of sight. It means believing that the missing pieces of our resources are not irrevocably gone, but instead lie deep inside our being, awaiting recovery.

Part of the binding-up process may involve getting professional counseling or therapy. Like the man of Bethesda, we sometimes can't make it into the healing waters on our own. Our relational wounds have so crippled us that we can no longer journey unaided. For the lame man of Bethesda, it took thirty-eight years to learn to walk again. His was not empty waiting. All the while, he watched for an opportunity that would bring him to the place where healing could happen.

Tending our broken hearts means having the courage of Peter to acknowledge the real places of our relational failures — where we know we have betrayed love, and all we can do is weep bitterly.

And, like Peter, it also means letting go of the guilt of our acknowledged mistakes and feeling worthy again to run to the place of resurrection.

The Oil of Gladness: Rituals for Healing

For the believing person, sacred ritual has always been associated with healing. Water. Oil. Garlands of flowers and words of blessing. The gifts of the earth and the proclamations of the heart can help us celebrate the growth that happens as we work toward psychosexual healing. Each of us needs to find the sacred symbols that for us ritualize both the ways we have already experienced new life and the hopes and expectations we hold for our continued movement toward relational health.

Rita is a young woman recovering from childhood sexual abuse and a failed marriage, who found her own special ritual after she began to heal the raw wounds of her own broken heart.

Lilacs have always had particular meaning for me. They're a sign of resilience against the harshness of winter and a hint of the beauty to come. Every spring, when the lilacs are in their first bloom, I pick several bunches of them and put them in vases all around my apartment. Then I fill the tub for a warm bath and float purple lilac blossoms all over the water. I put a little vial of lilac oil on the edge of the tub. Then I get in and let myself sink into the wonderful scent and feel of the warm water and the fresh blossoms. I image my body being caressed by beauty and gentleness. Then I take the lilac oil and I anoint all the places on my body that were hurt in the past. The places that were abused or treated roughly, I bless with tenderness. Each springtime when I celebrate my special ritual, I feel like I am returning, little by little, to the holy ground that is my body.

The Spirit of the Lord Yahweh has been given to me,
   ...to comfort all those who mourn and to give them for
      ashes a garland;
for mourning robe the oil of gladness...
                                        — Isaiah 61:1, 3

Long-term Effects of Psychosexual Wounds[18]

This table describes the long-term effects of wounds suffered at various stages of development.

CHILDHOOD

Phase I: Sexual Unawareness

1. These adults tend to be asexual — their interest in sexual thoughts, fantasies, feelings, or behaviors is limited or absent.

2. They may appear infantile or naive regarding sex.

3. They often have difficulty "feeling their feelings" in other areas of life.

4. They may tend to be dependent on others for nurturance.

Phase II: Sexual Awakening

1. Adults fixated here tend to behave inappropriately regarding sex. They are sexually awake but have not adequately socialized their heightened sexual interest.

2. They tend to be focused on themselves, may be attention seeking, often look for approval, and are easily threatened by others.

3. Relationships tend to be short term and lacking depth.

4. There is some evidence that adults who are more sexually interested in children than in adults are fixated here.

Phase III: Psychosexual Socialization

1. These adults tend to be secretly sexual. They think, feel, and act sexual, but are afraid to show it or talk about it.

2. They often have normal sexual feelings and fantasies, but, lacking adequate sexual information and too afraid to seek it directly, they may not know what is normal and what is not.

3. They may be outwardly very judgmental about the sexual behavior of others.

4. Being ultraprivate about themselves, they have difficulty with self-disclosure. Thus, they do not do well in relationships.

5. Some of these adults may obtain vicarious sexual enjoyment via romance novels, soap operas, and sexually explicit movies.

6. Individuals who have problems with compulsive masturbation or who use pornography as a primary form of sexual gratification are fixated here.

ADOLESCENCE

Phase I: Sexual Fantasizing

1. These adults limit their sexuality to the realm of fantasy. They derive more enjoyment from dreams than from reality.

2. They idealize relationships — so, they are usually disappointed in real life relationships. No one meets their expectations.

3. Jealousies, resentments, and conflicts tend to characterize their relationships. They are apt to be chronically possessive.

Phase II: Sexual Preoccupation

1. These adults are preoccupied with sex, as well as with themselves. Their focus on sexual imagery and self-enhancement often keeps them from enjoying deeper forms of sharing. They often behave as if their wants, needs, desires, and feelings are the only ones that count.

2. They tend to see people in terms of "body parts." Often they have minimal interest in relating to the real person inside the body.

3. Sex is the continual frame of reference for much of their thinking and valuing. (The characters "Sam" on the television sitcom "Cheers" and "Bea" on "Golden Girls" portray adults who are sexually fixated at the adolescent level of sexual preoccupation.)

4. Adults fixated here often use others and tend to end relationships that no longer please or excite them.

Phase III: Relational Exploration

1. These adults are usually superficial in their relationships. They are often fearful of being rejected, so they tend to be pleasers.

2. They are very sensitive to others' reactions to them, and often need more affirmation, support, and attention than do more secure adults.

3. Celibates who are fixated here tend to feel more comfortable with many friends and are hesitant to become invested in a single, close relationship. This can lead both to a scattered feeling, as well as to "love 'em and leave 'em" behaviors.

4. Adults fixated here still tend to make relational decisions on the basis of "what is best for me."

ADULTHOOD

Phase I: Psychosexual Mutuality

1. These adults are able to sustain healthy, mutual friendships, but they may tend to limit themselves to what feels safe, protective, or proper.

2. They may fear taking risks, standing alone, or tolerating normal relational tensions for long periods of time.

3. While generally healthy, these adults may be hesitant to engage in deeper, more intimate, affectionate, or vulnerable relationships, if such relationships feel at all threatening.

Phase II: Psychosexual Integration

There are no fixations here, only continual progression toward lifelong integration.

QUESTIONS FOR REFLECTION AND SHARING

These questions have been designed to help you personalize what you have just read. They are a way of getting in touch with your own story, of exploring what in you needs further growth or healing. Do not feel that you have to respond to all of them. Also, you may wish to reflect on them over several occasions. You may find it helpful to spend some time in prayer with them, to record your responses in your journal, or in some cases to share your responses with a close friend or significant other.

1. As you listen to your sexual story, where do you see evidence of sexual trauma? Punishment? Unhealthy guilt? Relational failure? Self-centeredness?

2. How have any of these experiences influenced your ability to enjoy relationships today? What have been their effects in your life? How do they "live on" in your relational style?

3. What have been your most embarrassing sexual moments? Frightening? Hurtful? How do these affect your ability to trust? Feel your feelings?

4. What have been your most life-giving sexual moments? Most freeing or healing? Most treasured? How have these nourished your relationships?

5. What part of your psychosexual history do you most regret? Do those regrets call you to any action today?

6. What most needs changing in your current mode of sexual thinking, behaving, or relating? Healing? Forgiving?

7. Is there any evidence in your life that your sexual energy is "on hold"? Imprisoned? Separated from your life? Fearful?

8. Are there any ways in which you have been (or still are) hurtful to others psychosexually? Used them? Been abusive, sexually, emotionally, or physically? If so, can you seek help?

9. If you have been sexually abused, have you had professional therapy for your abuse?

NOTE: Today "state of the art" treatment for sexual abuse requires that the therapist is registered or licensed by the state and has had extensive supervision in the treatment of sexual abuse. Just as an obstetrician would not be qualified to perform cardiac surgery, not all counselors, psychologists, psychiatrists, or group leaders are qualified to treat this most sensitive of conditions. Also, therapy prior to the last five to eight years may not have included more recent treatment advances. If you are seeking therapy for sexual abuse or malpractice, be sure that your therapist is licensed/registered and has had the required number of hours of supervision in sexual abuse treatment. Therapy for sexual abuse usually involves weekly sessions for an average of two or three years. While spiritual directors may provide important support and understanding to survivors of sexual abuse, they are not qualified to provide treatment — unless they are also licensed therapists who have had the required supervision.

10

I CALL YOU FRIENDS

Psychosexual Development and Human Intimacy

I shall not call you servants any more,
because a servant does not know his master's business;
   I call you friends,
because I have made known to you *everything*
I have learnt from my Father.

— John 15:15

It was a bittersweet moment. Jesus was telling his own closest friends how much he loved them. He was also saying goodbye. Here, we find him the way we usually do in John's gospel — lingering over the human. Saying out loud what is deepest in his heart. Being the Word. Making it flesh.

In his last hours, we don't find the Son of God on a hillside giving final admonitions to the crowds. We don't find him working one last miracle or preparing a defense for the religious officials who were opposed to him. Something of these last days gives us a clue about what was central to Jesus. He is at a meal with *his own* — a meal charged with the emotion of close friends parting. He is talking — talking about what is most significant to him, most worthy of remembering.

Be friends to each other in the same way that I have been a friend to you. I call you friends because I have *made known to you everything* . . . I've kept no secrets. I've hidden no emotion.

153

I Call You Friends. "Friend" was the word the author of John's gospel used to describe the relationship between Jesus and his closest disciples. There are two words in Greek that mean "friend" — hence, two different words John could have chosen to describe the friendship that existed between Jesus and his disciples. One of them, *hetairos*, means an associate or comrade. It suggests a level of relationship that involves familiarity, companionship, or sharing common concerns, but it does not indicate emotional closeness. John's gospel uses the second word, *philos*, which means "the beloved" or "dear one." Implying a deeper level of connection than *hetairos*, a *philos* assumes genuine love for the other. The relationship between Jesus and his closest disciples went beyond ordinary, friendly rapport to include real bonds of affection.

I call you *philos* — friend in the deepest, most loving sense of the word. To Jesus, those closest disciples were truly dear to him. They were his beloved ones. More than pupils learning rules, they shared his everything. More than co-workers or traveling companions, they held his heart. Implicit in the word is the assumption of self-disclosure. Jesus considered his disciples friends precisely because he had been able to share his everything with them.

Because I Have Made Known Everything.... We can over-spiritualize the content of the "everything" that Jesus shared with his friends at that meal. We can imagine him revealing divine truths, dictating doctrines, or summarizing his teachings to a group of obedient followers. Yet, to identify the "everything" of Jesus only with religious concepts is to miss the reality of his utter humanness. It is to make him a resident theologian instead of a friend.

The gospel accounts make it clear that Jesus spoke of religious truths. He gave his disciples a vision of the reign of God and emphasized the great commandment. Part of his "everything," then, involved instruction. But imparting information does not forge the bonds of friendship that *philos* suggests. Revealing great truths to attentive followers might equip them to preach the reign of God accurately, but it will not evoke the passion that enabled them to commit their hearts and lives to sustaining his memory for two thousand years. If "friend" describes the relationship between Jesus and his closest disciples, there was more shared than dogma. Religious truths might excite the intellect, but they rarely warm the soul. Friendship does not happen when I share information. It happens when I share my heart. Friendship is not a result of being in charge, but of being vulnerable.

Jesus knew some things about friendship. Although he did not use the language of modern psychology to describe it, he knew that self-disclosure was its most important ingredient — sharing his "everything." The gospels are filled with glimpses of Jesus the friend — Jesus engaged in transparent self-disclosure. His was a disclosure that surpassed the safe world of intellectual ideas and revealed the inner places of his most tender feelings and urgent needs:

> ... keep awake with me ... (Mt 26:38)

> ... Have I been with you so long, and yet you do not know me ...? (Jn 14:9)

> ... My soul is sorrowful to the point of death. (Mt 26:38)

> ... grieved at their hardness of heart, he looked angrily around at them ... (Mk 3:5)

> ... Jesus loved Martha and her sister and Lazarus ... (Jn 11:5)

> ... Jesus wept, and the Jews said, "See how much he loved him!" (Jn 11:35–36)

I call you friends, because I have made known to you "everything." Stay with me. We've been together so long. You don't understand me. My heart is aching. I have such deep longing. I'm angry. I want to be with you. I love you. I'm troubled. *Everything.*

Convictions about the reign of God? Yes. Laws articulated? Rules expounded? Disciplines urged? Of course. But that creates followers, not friends. True friendship was born of the stuff of the heart. The expression of feelings. The honest admission of needs. Tears cried in the open. Confrontations spoken out loud. Friendship was carved out of naming the doubts and sharing the dreams. It started at a lake and flowered in the ordinary places of life: in cornfields, at parties, on the road. It was cemented as words of affection were voiced and losses were grieved. It was tested in Gethsemane and denied in a courtyard. It survived misunderstandings and transcended fears. And through it all, it was self-disclosure — *making known everything* — that carried Jesus and his disciples from the teacher-student relationship to the warm ground of friendship.

Friendship doesn't happen simply because we share a common vision, engage in a mutual project, or spend time together. It is not an automatic by-product of living together, working with each other, playing golf, or taking a tour. Having sex neither produces nor sustains friendship by itself. Friendship happens because someone begins the arduous and sometimes painful, sometimes exhilarating work of self-disclosure, and invites the other to do the same.

Friendship and Sexuality

We have described sexuality as other-orienting energy. As such, sexuality prompts us to move toward one another. Its power urges us to become known in ever more progressive ways — to become psychologically naked. Psychological nakedness is to sexuality what physical nakedness is to genitality. Both invite the other to be naked — but each in a different way. Both have something to do with *philos*.

Physical nakedness involves taking one's clothes off — undressing the flesh, baring the body. Psychological nakedness involves taking one's masks off — undressing the heart, baring the soul. Ideally, in love relationships these two forms of nakedness go together. They are born to dance around each other in a gentle rhythm of gradually increasing vulnerability, transparency, and mutuality. When stories are shared and feelings are expressed, when hurts are tended and faults are made known without fear of reprisal, when tears do not have to be hidden and laughter is real, when angers are named and affection is honest, psychological nakedness is coming to birth.

While the fullest expression of human nakedness occurs when both psychological and physical forms are present, there may be instances when one occurs without the other. It is our belief that physical nakedness finds its deepest meaning when psychological nakedness is also part of the relationship. However, the opposite is not always true: psychological nakedness can be part of a relationship where sharing physical nakedness is either inappropriate or simply not desired. It can occur among:

- close friends

- business partners or co-workers

- members of support groups where self-disclosure is high

- parents and their adult children

- siblings or relatives

- engaged couples who are not sexually active

- celibate friends

In each of these instances, increasing levels of self-disclosure and emotional transparency can characterize the relationship. The critical factor is that mutuality and equality are present. As more of the inmost self of one person is revealed, it is met with reciprocal self-revelation on the part of the other. This ever-deepening psychological nakedness gives physical nakedness a context of love, if and when it is shared.

In our contemporary society, however, physical and psychological nakedness can easily become separated — especially among those who are too fearful to become emotionally vulnerable to one another. In such cases, removing clothing can become a substitute for removing one's emotional guard. The most extreme form of this behavior occurs in darkened houses and cheap motels, where insecure adolescents and lonely adults attempt to ease their pain by having sex — sometimes with people whose last names they don't know. In a society that often equates sex with intimacy, it is not surprising that relationally isolated individuals would attempt to find human closeness by genital contact devoid of interpersonal sharing.

The following example, recently told to us by a young graduate student, illustrates the common tendency to confuse genital activity with genuine intimacy:

I had been dating someone new, and I was telling a co-worker about it. She listened with interest as I described the things my date and I had been doing. But she grew impatient as I spoke of hiking, fireside conversations, and long walks by the lake. After a few minutes, she burst out asking, "Have you been intimate yet?" I knew she wasn't asking about the depth of our sharing. She wanted to know if we had been to bed.

Intimacy and Sexuality

Have you been intimate yet? We can look at this question on different levels. The story above illustrates one of them. At this level, intimacy is synonymous with genital experience. It implies having sex — being physically naked. It does not necessarily suggest anything more than that. At this level, there is no exchange of meaning, only an exchange of body fluids. Self-disclosure is not required. Neither is honesty, trust, caring, mutuality, or fidelity. When sex is over, so is "intimacy."

Even though it may not sound fulfilling, this kind of "intimacy" has considerable following in our western culture. At all levels of society we can find people who believe — or behave as though they believe — that the purpose of sex is physical enjoyment with whatever partner seems exciting at the time. At this level, sex is variously considered a way of getting to know someone, a way of easing loneliness, or simply a way to have a good time.

It is not only the lonely, the promiscuous, the advocates of free love and anonymous sex who involve themselves in such minimal levels of "intimacy." Actually, it can also be found in committed relationships of some duration. There are more than a few married couples who, day after day, sit at the same table, drive the same car, share the same bank account, rear the same children, and sleep in the same bed whose sexual sharing portrays a level of intimacy that goes no deeper than the perfunctory genital contact characteristic of people who hardly know each other. Self-disclosure cannot be presumed by virtue of a marriage certificate. Physical nakedness, even when shared for years with the same partner, does not automatically blossom into psychological nakedness. It is a sad reality that many married people live their entire lives with occasional sexual intercourse as their only form of intimacy — their only way of being naked with each other. Whether among married couples, good-time seekers, or isolated drifters, when intimacy is equated with having sex, little more is shared than an orgasm and a few minutes of physical closeness.

What happens when we see intimacy in the context of human experience and committed faith? Genuine intimacy, in its most profound sense, may be likened to *philos* — the friendship described in John's gospel. Intimacy involves making known our *everything* to a dear one. It is experienced gradually and deepens slowly as mutual self-disclosure increases. While genuine affection may be present early, sex is reserved for a later stage of the relationship — if and when it is chosen. The emphasis is on psychological nakedness — progressive revelation of the inmost self.

Genuine intimacy does not develop quickly or easily. It grows slowly as stories are shared. It deepens as the other is invited to peek into the secret crevices and sometimes hidden places of our lives. Ever so slowly, our pretenses of perfection slip away. Sometimes haltingly, we let our guard down and the less attractive parts of our personalities and histories are invited into the daylight. No longer trying to impress the other with an unblemished self, our defenses, protections, and masks increasingly give way to truth.

Intimacy. Friendship. Love. The true self revealed. Somewhere in the deep recesses of our beings, we all hunger for it — the hunger is built into us from the beginning. So is the energy to seek it. We call it sexuality.

The emotions of friendship that sear our hearts are as familiar to us as they were to Jesus. How often have we looked out over the city or the countryside and felt longing surge up in our beings to hold or be held, to comfort or be comforted? How often have we tasted the bitter disappointment of being with someone, perhaps for a long time, who still does not really know us on the inside? How often have we spilled out tears that couldn't be choked back because someone we love is gone? How often has a dear one filled our hearts with so much love that we could hardly find words to describe it or a place in our bodies to contain it?

We know the emotions of friendship well. They are the driving energies behind our efforts to find each other. Taken together, the emotions of friendship and the behaviors of self-disclosure converge in the one great energy of sexuality. It is our sexual energy that urges us, if we are healthy, to orient ourselves toward those whose very existence lights fire in our flesh and puts welcome in our eyes. It is our sexual energy that invites us to approach, to seek out, to open up, to receive, to forgive, to be faithful. It is our sexual energy that carries us away from isolation and toward one another. It is an awesome energy, a terrible power. It can hurt as well as help. It can abuse as well as care.

Have You Been Intimate Yet?

It is a haunting question. Have you shared your *everything* yet? Have you told your life stories to someone and listened as they told theirs? Have you let your guard down with anyone yet? Have you taken off your masks and gently peeled away the many layers of protection that hide your true self with some-one, somewhere, sometime? Have you sobbed unashamed in someone's arms and held them as they wept? Have you felt their sadness in your bones and recognized it as yours as well? Have you been giddy and silly with someone, just because you felt so free in their presence? Have you whispered your darkest secrets and spoken of your wildest dreams with anyone — yet?

Intimacy has to do with behaviors — actions that enable us to connect with each other. We define intimacy as *loving behavior that is manifested through self-disclosure*. Let's look at this definition of intimacy in greater detail.

The word "intimacy" is derived from two Latin words — *intimus* (inside of) and *intimidare* (to fear or be in awe). The Latin roots point up the ambiguity that often surrounds our experiences with intimacy. Being close enough to be *inside of* another — or to let another inside us — is at once awesome and fearsome. It both draws and repels, pulls us in and pushes us back. It fills us with wonder and scares us at the same time. The very thing we all seek — close human connection — can also be very intimidating. It demands that we let go of con-trol and give up the safety of our solitariness. It requires a

journey into the often unchartered waters of relationship —
where there are no maps, no guarantees, and even less cer-
tainty about the ultimate destination. It is a journey that can
be at once exhilarating and terrifying, exhausting and nour-
ishing. The more we enter "inside of" the life of another and
allow that person to do the same with us, the more we are
in the space where strength and fragility live alongside each
other. Nowhere can pain burn so deeply or joy penetrate so
totally as in a relationship where *intimus* and *intimidare* are
etching their portraits into our hearts.

Eventually, the movement toward the other must gain mo-
mentum over the urge to pull away. The desire to be intimate
must carry us past the fears and inadequacies that stare us in
the face. As genuine closeness becomes a possibility, we may
need to fight the desire to run and hide. Otherwise, we will
stay irrevocably locked in ambiguity. Immobilized by the fears
of intimacy, yet drawn into its embrace, we can become like
a phonograph record stuck in one place — doomed to repeat
one line of a song until the electricity is cut off and the music
dies.

There are people who live their whole lives like this. They
are afraid to follow through with radical self-disclosure after
the initial foray into connection with another. When they feel
the heat of a growing closeness, they either end a relationship
or they play the game of psychological "catch me if you can."
The rules of the game are simple: Just throw out enough hints
of the true self to keep the other person from leaving, but don't
let them get too close. Be interesting without being vulnerable.
Tease or flirt, but don't risk genuine self-disclosure. Take your
clothes off, but keep your soul tightly wrapped.

It isn't easy to invite another person into our hearts or to
tread the path into another's deepest self. It is far easier to take
our clothes off than it is to take our masks off. Stepping out
of our garments asks much less of us than stepping out from
behind the barriers of self-protection that we have so carefully
erected. A night of physical closeness and a few moments of
pelvic pleasure are much less arduous than months and years
of mutual self-disclosure.

Intimus. Inside of.... The physical images of mutual inter-
penetration are as familiar as they are beautiful — two persons

whose flesh becomes one as their bodies and hearts unite. Even if this experience has not been personalized in our own lives, novels, movies, and our capacity for fantasy and imagination can help us picture it. In contrast, the images of emotional, spiritual intercoursing are not as obvious to us or as easy to picture.

Most of us can visualize two people kissing, caressing, having sex. It is more difficult — and certainly less titillating — to call up images of these same people sitting at a kitchen table in tears, trying desperately to find each other after an argument. It would be far more enjoyable to let them tell us fairy tales and take us to never-never-land, than to allow them to remind us that "happily-ever-after" comes with a price, if it comes at all.

Telling the Stories

Once upon a time — why are these words more familiar to children than to adults? It is, after all, we adults whose lives carry more stories; we've had more years to create them. Even more ironic, while children listen with rapt attention to the tales of Cinderella and Robin Hood, we can hear the music at the ball and smell the dampness of the forest. We've lived long enough by now to have been there. To us, the search for acceptance and the struggle to overcome evil are no longer make believe.

It is our stories more than anything else that provide us with the key building blocks of intimacy. It is in telling all the stories our life holds — gradually, mutually — that true intimacy happens. Soul nakedness unfolds. Then, as in a well-orchestrated liturgy, our stories mingle with celebration. When the psyche is as naked to the other as is the body, we have sacred ritual. Holy rites.

Intimacy is not for the fainthearted. It is not for those who need to control their relationships with others. Nor is it for those whose requirements for personal privacy outweigh their willingness or their ability to tolerate exposure of the mystery that defines their "inmost self."

Intimacy is for everyday folks who are afraid of being rejected, but even more afraid of being alone. It is for the hesitant and the faltering, whose insufficiencies and failures have made them a little more sensitive to others and a little more aware of themselves. It is for those who feel awkward with vulnerability, but still choose it over the chill of inter-personal distance. It is for those who sometimes have a hard time expressing their feelings, but who keep searching for the words just the same. It is for people who know the phrases that sustain intimacy and try to say them, at least some of the time: I'm sorry. I don't know. I need you. Stay with me. For-give me. I'm threatened. I'm angry. You mean so much to me. I love you.

I love you. These poignant words reveal another aspect of intimacy: Genuine intimacy involves *love*. Our behavior must enable another to feel our care, our concern, our respect. It is not sufficient to act unreflectively in a relationship where I desire closeness. Love must be articulated in my actions.

Loving behavior refers not only to the romantic love we might have for a spouse or significant other, but also to the affection and care we have toward any person who is close to us — a parent, a child, a sibling, a good friend. It is this love that Jesus expressed for his own in John's gospel. Love is revealed in tender words and in the honest admission of feelings. It holds the other dear. It wishes for nearness and never wants to be forgotten: Love one another. Don't let your hearts be troubled. Trust in me. I'm preparing a place for you. We'll be separated for awhile and that will be hard. Believe in me. I'll do as much as I can for you. I won't leave you. Don't leave me either. I'm telling you this now so you will be prepared for what lies ahead. I don't want anyone to take away your joy. I call you friends because I've told you everything I know.

Loving behavior that is manifested takes more than silent devotion, more than quiet concern, to fill out the portrait of intimacy. Our actions of love must live in the light. They must be shown, articulated, demonstrated so those we love can feel them. Do you love me? It was the question asked by Tevye's wife of twenty-five years in the musical "Fiddler on the Roof." Do you love me? How sad to be married that long and need to ask such a question. Sadder still was his response: "Do I love you? After twenty-five years, I suppose I do." Some of Tevye's inability to make his love verbally manifest to his wife can be understood in light of the arranged marriages of the time. People did not marry for love, so it is understandable that they would not give it much conscious thought over the years. Eventually, Tevye and his wife discovered their love. Though words of love had never been exchanged, there were other manifestations of it in their relationship. It was the words, however, that brought the quiet wondering into the open. It was the words that were missing — words that eventually need to be spoken when intimacy is at stake. Loving behavior that is manifested. To experience intimacy, we need to see it, feel it, touch it, hear it. It has to get through to us as a living, breathing reality that eases our wondering and relieves our questions about the depth of our connections to others.

Intimacy is loving behavior manifested in self-disclosure.

I call you friends because I have made known to you everything.

These are two different ways of saying essentially the same thing. One uses the language of psychology and provides a neat definition. It comes from the laboratories of behavioral research. The other uses a biblical story and offers us an image. It comes from a table conversation after a meal. But both are talking about revealing the inmost self to a dear one, the beloved. Both are stressing the importance of unveiling the self in the context of significant relationships. Both suggest that the pathway to intimacy unfolds as the heart is revealed — that friendship becomes a possibility when my *everything* is made known.

Intimacy vs. Intimate Experiences

There are some relationships that provide an intimate experience for one person and not for the other. Something intimate happens, but it is not mutual. One person is experiencing a level of self-revelation or vulnerability and the other is not. This is the case when one person is providing a service for another, or when the experience is occurring among people who do not have equal power or influence in the relationship. Examples include:

- Parents and children
- Teachers and students
- Therapist and client
- Spiritual director and directee
- Physician and patient

In each of these cases, one person is more vulnerable and has less power by virtue of that vulnerability. For the woman who is having a pelvic examination, the experience for her is an intimate one. It is not intimate for the doctor. The same is true for a client who reveals a painful history of sexual abuse to his therapist. It would be not only inappropriate but a violation of professional ethics for the therapist to talk about his past sexual abuse in the hope of finding some support from his client. In the same way, parents are in a position of protection and care in relationship to their children. Even though there are close ties and affectional bonds between them, full equality, in terms of equal power sharing, is not present.

Whenever we are involved in relationships where one person is identified as a helper or a resource, mutuality and equality are not proportionate. Consequently, friendship and genuine intimacy are not a possibility. Even though some of the characteristics of intimacy might be present, mutual self-disclosure, the bedrock of intimacy, is not.

Love One Another

> I give you a new commandment: love one another; just as I have loved you, you also must love one another. By this love you have for one another, everyone will know that you are my disciples.
>
> — John 13:34–35

All believers are called to make love. For those of us who claim to follow the God who gave us the great commandment, intimacy is not an option, it's a necessity. Engaging in self-disclosure, making known *my everything*, are not choices in the smorgasbord of Christian living. I cannot profess to follow the gospel and then decide that self-revelation is not for me. I cannot present myself as one of the disciples of Jesus of Nazareth and opt to live my life outside of relationships. Love happens in the midst of human contact. It is more than a benevolent act of the mind that wishes someone well. It shows in our eyes. It is heard in our tone of voice. It is felt in our touch. And that is how *everyone will know*. . . .

We have so many ways to make love. Perhaps the most obvious is having physical sex. But we can make love with our words, with our eyes, with our sensitive care for one another. Each time we interpenetrate our hearts, each time we say what we honestly think and feel in a way that honors and respects the beloved, each time we exchange some part of our *everything* with a dear one, we are making love.

Sexuality is an integral part of our many forms of love-making. Its cosmic fire is always with us as embodied male or female persons. Our sexual energy is revealed via facial animation, eye contact, tone of voice, expressions of affection, communication, and body posture. When it is operative, we seem alive, dynamic, and emotionally present. When it is not, there is a sense of emotional vacuity, of distance, coldness, or aloofness about us. In the absence of sexual energy, it might seem that there is a body there without a person inside. The body moves, talks, and breathes, but offers no possibility of a relational connection. Sexual energy is like an electrical charge in the air. We are warmed by its varying degrees of intensity or chilled by its absence.

Sexuality. Friendship. Intimacy. Making love. We have been weaving all these words around each other, offering images, and examining definitions, but we have not made clear distinctions between them. Each of us has our own perceptions of what these words mean in our own lives. It is not our desire to provide fixed definitions for these most personal of human experiences.

The Many Faces of Making Love

Making love is the activity of intimacy, the expression of *philos*. It is what we do with our beloved, our dear ones, whenever we reveal our inmost selves. Some good friends of many years — we will call them Mary and Jim — shared this true story of their lovemaking with us.

Mary and Jim had been married almost ten years. They had both felt some gradual distance creeping into their relationship as the years went by. It didn't seem very serious, but quietly worrisome just the same.

Although they felt they had a good marriage, both of them had the unspoken feeling that the romance was gone from their relationship. They had three young children, active careers, and an ever expanding list of meetings, obligations, and friends. There was very little time for them just to be alone with each other, much less to share their feelings at any depth.

As they discussed what they would do to celebrate, they concluded that they needed to rekindle the wonderful romance that had characterized the first years of their marriage. They made a reservation for the bridal suite at a luxurious hotel on the weekend of their tenth anniversary, which was three months away. They began readying themselves for the event. To do so, they each focused on enhancing the physical aspects of their relationship.

With each of their children Mary had gained an extra ten pounds that she never lost. Her hair seemed lifeless, and she had a chipped front tooth that she thought made her less attractive. Jim was equally out of shape, with an emerging potbelly and sagging biceps. He had a mustache when they married and had shaved it off years ago. He resolved to grow it back — perhaps it would remind Mary of the way he looked when they first met.

As the weeks went by, their anticipation grew. Mary joined an aerobics class and got her tooth fixed. Jim pumped iron and took up jogging. His mustache made its appearance and he felt quite dashing. Mary got her hair highlighted. A few weeks before the magic weekend, she bought a lovely negligee. By the time the anniversary date arrived, they were ready.

After giving last-minute instructions to the babysitter, they drove to their romantic hideaway and checked in for the weekend. Their accommodations were exquisite — a heart-shaped bed, a heart-shaped jacuzzi, and a heart-shaped basket filled with flowers and champagne. That evening they enjoyed a romantic candlelight dinner by the pool. Afterward they went for a long walk in the moonlight and kissed and caressed in the hotel garden like young lovers. Even the weather was celebrating with them. Later, they took a bath in their jacuzzi, then gave each other a tender massage. They made love. Eventually, their heart-shaped bed carried them to sleep.

Then something mysterious happened. About 4:00 a.m. Mary woke up crying — she wasn't sure why. Jim was awakened by her sobs. "What's wrong? Are you all right? Was it something I said? Wasn't . . . wasn't it good for you?" he queried anxiously.

"No, it isn't that — last night was wonderful. I don't know — I feel so strange, so alone or something, . . ." Mary replied between gulps. They held each other. They started to talk about Mary's feeling of aloneness; Jim acknowledged that he sometimes felt it too. They talked of their fragility, their fears of losing each other. They spoke of their doubts and wondered out loud if each was still attractive to the other. Jim found his own tears as he told Mary how he sometimes worried that she wished she had married her old boyfriend from high school. He had always been too afraid or too proud to ask her before. They reassured each other, half crying and half laughing. They talked of death and of what it would be like to be left if the other died first. They named some old angers that they had never been able to bring out in the open. They spoke words of forgiveness and words of hope for the future. There, in the night, with morning breath and rumpled hair, they talked and laughed, and cried together as the hours passed unnoticed. Before they knew it, dawn gave way to morning. It was 7:00 a.m. It had been years since they had talked for so many hours while time stood still. They knew then they would make it. They were still in love.

Mary and Jim had made love around midnight. Their physical sex took place in the context of their shared history. Over the years, they had loved each other well and been happy together. They had engaged in periodic self-disclosure, and their intimacy was deeply rooted and secure. But this night of nights, something special happened for them. They learned something about making love — something old and something new — something that they each had known in their hearts and even experienced, yet something fresh and young at the same time. It was this: Genital sex can be a wondrous experience of sharing. But when physical nakedness flows from and celebrates the psychological nakedness that has already taken place on another level, intimacy is complete and making love is even more exhilarating.

Making love. Experiencing intimacy. We do it whenever we stay awake long into the night sharing stories with a friend while time stands still. We do it when we laugh until our sides hurt with someone close. We do it when we cry in one another's arms, because the conflict that always comes with intimacy can hurt so much. And we do it whenever we say to someone who holds our heart: I call you friend because I have made known to you everything.

QUESTIONS FOR REFLECTION AND SHARING

These questions have been designed to help you personalize what you have just read. They are a way of getting in touch with your own story, of exploring what in you needs further growth or healing. Do not feel that you have to respond to all of them. Also, you may wish to reflect on them over several occasions. You may find it helpful to spend some time in prayer with them, to record your responses in your journal, or in some cases to share your responses with a close friend or significant other.

1. What qualities seem to characterize your relationships with others? What is your behavior like in relationships?

2. Can you name one or more very close friends — where mutuality is present?

3. Who knows your heart? With whom can you cry? Confide your deepest feelings?

4. As you look over the history of your adult relationships, what do you see in terms of permanence of relationships? Fidelity? Managing conflict? Mutual satisfaction with the relationship?

5. With what kinds of people have your relationships been stormy? Unsatisfying? What role did you play in the problem? What role did they play?

6. To what degree are you controlling in relationships? Passive? Critical? Jealous?

7. To what degree are you encouraging? Sharing? Positive? Supportive?

8. What did you learn about how to be a friend from your parents? How do your relationships today reflect theirs? How are yours different?

9. Is there something you need to say to someone who is important to you that you have been unable or afraid to say?

10. How effective are your communication skills? Your ability to know, name, and express your feelings appropriately?

NOTES

1 / Cosmic Allurement

1. Stephen W. Hawking, *A Brief History of Time: From the Big Bang to Black Holes* (Toronto: Bantam Books, 1988), 70–71.

2. Brian Swimme, *The Universe Is a Green Dragon* (Santa Fe: Bear & Co., 1985), 43–52.

3. Ibid., 49.

4. John Paul II, *On the Family (Familiaris Consortio)*, Apostolic Exhortation, December 15, 1981, see no. 11.

5. Jean Houston, *The Search for the Beloved: Journeys in Mythology and Sacred Psychology* (Los Angeles: Jeremy P. Tarcher, 1987); see especially 24–25, 143–45.

2 / A Future With Hope

6. Alice Walker, *The Color Purple* (New York: Simon & Schuster Pocket Books, 1982), 203.

3 / Pathway to Love

7. Sacred Congregation for the Doctrine of the Faith, *Declaration on Certain Questions Concerning Sexual Ethics*, December 29, 1975, no. 1.

8. United States Catholic Conference, *Human Sexuality: A Catholic Perspective for Education and Lifelong Learning* (Washington, D.C.: USCC Publications, 1991).

9. The original schema for this stage approach to psychosexual development was developed by Michael E. Cavanaugh, Ph.D., in an article entitled "The Impact of Psychosexual Growth on Marriage and Religious Life," *Human Development* 4 (Fall 1983), 16–24. We have modified and further elaborated some of his ideas, but we are indebted to Dr. Cavanaugh for his initial insights.

10. In a document entitled *Educational Guidance in Human Love* (November 1, 1983), the Congregation for Catholic Education states that chastity "consists in self-control, in the capacity of guiding the sexual instinct to the service of love and of integrating it in the development of the person."

4 / Knit Together in My Mother's Womb

11. Thomas Verny, M.D., *The Secret Life of the Unborn Child* (New York: Dell, 1981), 41.

12. William Masters and Virginia Johnson, *Masters & Johnson on Sex and Human Loving* (Boston: Little, Brown, 1988), 124.

13. Pope John Paul II, as quoted by Chet Raymo, "Stephen Hawking and the Mind of God," *Commonweal* 117, no. 7 (April 6, 1990), 220.

14. Pope Pius XII, address given to a group of Catholic obstetricians and gynecologists, January 8, 1956, in *Love and Sexuality: Official Catholic Teachings*, ed. Odile M. Liebard (Wilmington, N.C.: McGrath Publishing Co., 1978), 168.

7 / Coming Into Our Own

15. Peter Marin, "A Revolution's Broken Promises," *Psychology Today* (July 1983), 50–57.

8 / Seasons of the Heart

16. Judith Viorst, *Necessary Losses* (New York: Fawcett Gold Medal, 1986), 3.

17. Ibid., 2.

9 / To Bind Up Hearts That Are Broken

18. This outline is based on the summary given by Michael E. Cavanaugh, Ph.D., in "The Impact of Psychosexual Growth on Marriage and Religious Life," *Human Development* 4 (Fall 1983), 22–23.

SELECT BIBLIOGRAPHY

Human Sexuality: General

Gagnon, John H. *Human Sexualities*. Glenview, Ill.: Scott, Foresman, and Company, 1977.

Masters, William H., Virginia E. Johnson, and Robert C. Kolodny. *Masters and Johnson on Sex and Human Loving*. (Revised). Boston: Little, Brown, & Co., 1988.

Reinisch, June, Ph.D. *The Kinsey Institute New Report on Sex*. New York: St. Martin's Press, 1990.

Verny, Thomas, M.D., with John Kelly. *The Secret Life of the Unborn Child*. New York: Dell Publishing Co., 1981.

Sexuality and Spirituality

Catholic Theological Society of America (C.T.S.A.). *Human Sexuality: New Directions in Catholic Thought*. Ramsey, N.J.: Paulist Press, 1977.

Declaration on Certain Questions Concerning Sexual Ethics. Rome: Congregation of the Doctrine of the Faith, January 22, 1975.

Ferder, Fran, and John Heagle. *Partnership: Women and Men in Ministry*. Notre Dame: Ave Maria Press, 1989.

Koch, Carl, and Joyce Heil. *Created in God's Image: Meditating on Our Body*. Winona, Minn.: St. Mary's Press, 1991.

Nelson, James B. *Embodiment: An Approach to Sexuality and Christian Theology*. Minneapolis: Augsburg Press, 1978.

————. *Between Two Gardens: Reflections on Sexuality and Religious Experience*. New York: Pilgrim Press, 1987.

Trible, Phyllis. *God and the Rhetoric of Sexuality*. Philadelphia: Fortress Press, 1978.

173

United States Catholic Conference. *Human Sexuality: A Catholic Perspective for Education and Lifelong Learning*. Washington, D.C.: USCC Publications, 1991.

Male/Female Sexuality

Bly, Robert. *Iron John: A Book about Men*. Reading, Mass.: Addison-Wesley Publishing Co., 1990.

Carr, Anne E. *Transforming Grace: Christian Tradition and Women's Experience*. San Francisco: Harper & Row, 1990.

Cavanaugh, Michael E., Ph.D. "The Impact of Psychosexual Growth on Marriage and Religious Life," *Human Development* 4 (Fall 1983), 16–24.

McGill, Michael. *The McGill Report on Male Intimacy*. New York: Holt, Rinehart & Winston, 1985.

Sexuality and Celibacy

Clark, Keith. *Being Sexual and Celibate*. Notre Dame: Ave Maria Press, 1986.

Goergen, Donald. *The Sexual Celibate*. New York: The Seabury Press, 1974.

Huddleston, Mary Anne. *Celibate Loving*. Ramsey, N.J.: Paulist Press, 1984.

Sexuality and Marriage

Greeley, Andrew M. *Faithful Attraction: Discovering Intimacy, Love, and Fidelity in American Marriage*. New York: TOR Books, 1991.

Stehura, Eugene. *Love Talk: A Communication Guide for Married Couples*. Kansas City, Mo.: Sheed & Ward, 1991.

Whitehead, Evelyn Eaton, and James D. Whitehead. *Marrying Well: Stages on the Journey of Christian Marriage*. Garden City, N.Y.: Doubleday Image Books, 1983.

Sexual Orientation

Boswell, John. *Christianity, Social Tolerance, and Homosexuality*. Chicago: University of Chicago Press, 1980.

Gramick, Jeannine, ed. *Homosexuality and the Catholic Church*. Mt. Rainier, Md.: New Ways Ministry, 1983.

Scanzoni, Letha, and Virginia Ramey Mollenkott. *Is the Homosexual My Neighbor?* San Francisco: Harper & Row, 1978.

Sexual Abuse and Malpractice

Bass, Ellen, and Laura Davis. *The Courage to Heal: A Guide for Women Survivors of Child Sexual Abuse.* New York: Harper & Row, 1988.
Gill, Eliana, Ph.D. *Outgrowing the Pain: A Book for and About Adults Abused as Children.* New York: Dell Publishing, 1983.
Hunter, Mic. *Abused Boys: Neglected Victims of Sexual Abuse.* Lexington, Mass.: D. C. Heath and Company, 1990.